Host Defenses in the Human Neonate

Monographs in Neonatology

Thomas K. Oliver, Jr., M.D.
Series Editor

ANTIMICROBIAL THERAPY FOR NEWBORNS: PRACTICAL
APPLICATION OF PHARMACOLOGY TO CLINICAL USE
by George H. McCracken, Jr., M.D., and John D. Nelson, M.D.

TEMPERATURE REGULATION AND ENERGY METABOLISM IN
THE NEWBORN
by John C. Sinclair, M.D.

PERINATAL COAGULATION
by William E. Hathway, M.D., and John Bonnar, M.D.

Host Defenses
in the Human Neonate

by

Michael E. Miller, M.D.

Research Professor of Immunology
Chief, Division of Immunology and Hematology-Oncology
Department of Pediatrics
University of California, Los Angeles
School of Medicine
Harbor General Hospital Campus
Torrance, California

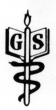

Grune & Stratton
A Subsidiary of Harcourt Brace Jovanovich, Publishers
NEW YORK   SAN FRANCISCO   LONDON

Library of Congress Cataloging in Publication Data

Miller, Michael E.
    Host defenses in the human neonate.

    Includes bibliographical references and index.
    1. Infection in children—Immunological
aspects.   2. Infants (Newborn)—Diseases—
Immunological aspects.   3. Immunology, Develop-
mental.   4. Immunological deficiency syndromes.
I. Title. [DNLM: 1. Immunity—In infancy and
childhood.   2. Infant, Newborn.   QW504.3 M649h]
RJ275.M54   618.9'201   78-18170
ISBN 0-8089-1094-9

Grune & Stratton, Inc.
111 Fifth Avenue
New York, New York 10003

Distributed in the United Kingdom by
Academic Press, Inc. (London) Ltd.
24/28 Oval Road, London NW 1

Library of Congress Catalog Number 78-18170
International Standard Book Number 0-8089-1094-9
Printed in the United States of America

To Paula, Carrie, Lisa, Rick,
and Jamie

Contents

Foreword

For this volume in the series of Monographs in Neonatology, Dr.
Michael Miller has undertaken the gargantuan task of writing
the entire book by himself! He is thoroughly equipped to do this
because he has been involved in studies of the host defenses of the
human neonate for a number of years.

A review of the table of contents reveals the comprehensive approach Miller has given to this important area of neonatology.
Here the interested reader will find a thorough discussion of the
development of the T-cell and B-cell systems, of phagocytic cells
and humoral mediators, as well as a description of various clinical
disorders of host defense. This volume represents a splendid addition to the series for which Dr. Miller is to be congratulated.

THOMAS K. OLIVER, JR., M.D.
Series Editor

Preface

The mechanisms by which the human fetus and newborn acquire resistance to infections are an area of immense biologic significance. Increased understanding of the ontogeny and interaction of these processes should provide all physicians involved in the care of newborns with important information for both the prevention of intra-uterine infections and management of their resultant sequelae—congenital malformations, growth dysfunctions, and mental retardation. This information also should aid in the development of improved therapy of neonatal septicemia, which remains a leading cause of infant morbidity and mortality. Characterization of the neonatal immune-inflammatory response provides the immunologist and developmental biologist with major tools by which to characterize the normal adult immune-inflammatory response. In this sense, the newborn is the ultimate "experiment of nature," providing the researcher with a rich store of naturally occurring maturational deficiencies through which normal immunologic functions can be probed.

In the last 20 years much information has accumulated which dispels the previous notion of the "immunologically null" infant. This book is a comprehensive review of this important information. Rather than deal with the subject from the traditional point of view of isolated systems of immunity, it approaches the topic from the point of view of host defenses, examining the interactions of the components of the inflammatory and immune responses.

MICHAEL E. MILLER

Acknowledgment

As with most books, this one could not have been written without the inspiration, guidance, and encouragement provided by many others. The immense help of Ms. Sue Sestich in assembling the material was critical in completion of the task.

1
General Concepts

A PHILOSOPHY OF NEONATES AND INFECTIONS

Those who read this book likely share the knowledge that newborn infants get more infections than is their due. Further, the infected neonate does not always make his or her plight obvious. Clinical signs are apt to be meager at best, and the physician caring for the afflicted infant is usually faced with an incomplete diagnostic picture.

Modern neonatal medicine has attempted to respond to these problems by seemingly logical approaches—focusing upon improved diagnostic and support measures and, in particular, upon specific antimicrobial therapy. Surprisingly, however, these measures have proven relatively ineffective in decreasing the mortality and morbidity of neonatal septicemia over the past four decades. This means that either the right combination of diagnosis, support, and antimicrobials has not yet been found or another set of mechanisms may be involved.

This book is concerned with the latter probability. As we shall see, the normal neonate exhibits numerous deficiencies in responses to infectious challenge. In describing these deficiencies, it is hoped to establish the primary importance of impaired host defenses in the neonate as a cause of the clinical abnormalities of infection characteristic of this period of life. It is not implied that antimicrobial therapy is unimportant but rather that definitive solutions are unlikely to result without enhancement of immune-inflammatory processes.

In support of this philosophy, it is useful to review some of the immunologic implications of established data on neonatal infections.

Microorganisms Involved in Neonatal Septicemia

Over the past four decades, there have been several shifts in the specific microorganisms predominately responsible for neonatal septicemia.[1,2] These have involved the group A beta-hemolytic streptococcus (1930s and 1940s), a phage group I *Staphylococcus aureus* (1950s), and *Escherichia coli* and the group B beta-hemolytic streptococci (late 1950s to present). The group B streptococci are presently the most common etiologic agents isolated from infants with septicemia and/or meningitis.[1] In vitro, none of these organisms are particularly difficult to eradicate. The group B streptococci, for example, are highly sensitive to a number of common antibiotics. Further, when encountered in a normal adult or older child, each of these organisms is relatively easy to treat with antimicrobials. It is only in the neonate that clinical difficulties are encountered.

One interpretation of this paradox would be that the neonate provides a special problem in distribution and tissue levels of antibiotics. Although there may be some truth in this hypothesis, there is little hard data to support it.

An alternative explanation is that the neonate lacks the full complement of mature immune-inflammatory processes necessary to combat infections effectively. It is interesting to note that patients with immunodeficiency disorders also have a high predilection for infections with organisms that in the normal subject would readily yield to therapy. Thus, frequent infections with organisms susceptible to antibiotics are characteristic of impaired host defenses.

Clinical Response to Infections

A number of signs and symptoms commonly occur in the normal patient with infection. Systemic findings may include fever, toxicity, chills, leukocytosis, and in CNS infections, meningeal signs. Local infections are usually characterized by pain, swelling, erythema, and warmth.

As every medical student is taught, the normal neonate is unlikely to show these findings. Fever, general toxicity, leukocytosis, and meningeal signs are seldom marked, and local infections rarely produce common inflammatory signs. Thus the neonate gives further evidence of an inappropriate response to infection. It is reasonable to assume that this hyporesponsiveness is a contributing factor in increased susceptibility to infections during the neonatal period.

Persistence of Viral Infections

Several viruses produce a unique picture when acquired during the perinatal period. For example, rubella or cytomegalovirus[3] may produce a persistent infection lasting for years, resulting in persistent antigen production. Similar persistence of viruses in older children and adults occurs but is rare. Although the molecular events underlying this phenomenon in the neonate are incompletely understood, there is evidence that immune complexes of different sizes may form during the course of congenital cytomegalovirus infections.[3] In early life, when the infections are asymptomatic, 13S complexes are primarily formed, while heavier 19 to 20S complexes are formed when the antigenic load increases. Stagno and co-workers have suggested that these heavier complexes may directly damage tissues and contribute to weakened host defenses.[3] If true, this would suggest that neonatal host defense mechanisms are more susceptible to such damage than host defense mechanisms of older children and adults. Alternatively, impaired host defense mechanisms may result in a different pattern of immune complex formation in neonates than in adults. Regardless of which explanation proves correct, the implication of impaired host defense mechanisms as a clinically significant contributing factor to neonatal infections is again underscored.

Improved Resistance to Infection in Immunologically Amplified Neonates

Although a detailed analysis is outside the scope of this book, the reader should be reminded of emerging data suggesting that breast-fed infants may have reduced frequency of infections[4-6] resulting from acquisition of maternal T cells, B cells, and macrophages.[4-7] Reduced frequencies of K1 positive *E. coli* meningitis and necrotizing enterocolitis have been observed in breast-fed infants.[4-6] Such data indirectly support the significance of impaired host defenses as a primary factor in neonatal infections.

The above examples indicate why study of host defenses of the neonate has become a particularly intriguing challenge to the pediatric immunologist. Better characterization of these mechanisms should lead not only to improved detection, diagnosis, and management of infected neonates but also to increased understanding of the normal immune response. In a sense, the neonate represents the ultimate "experiment of nature."

Before proceeding with detailed descriptions of the various components of host defenses, it is appropriate to outline the general areas encompassed by this term.

HOST DEFENSES: HISTORICAL AND GENERAL PERSPECTIVES

The concept of "host defenses" is a natural derivative of the truly remarkable progress made in the fields of clinical and basic immunology over the past 25 years. Through the discovery and dissection of naturally occurring abnormalities of the immune-inflammatory response, it has become apparent that resistance to infections in man involves a complex set of interactions.

The first such defect, or "experiment of nature," was described by Colonel Ogden Bruton, an Army pediatrician, in 1952.[8] Bruton studied a male child afflicted with repeated, severe bacterial infections who was relatively unresponsive to conventional antibiotic therapy. In the course of extensive evaluations over a number of years, Bruton discovered by serum electrophoresis that the patient lacked discernible immunoglobulins. He concluded that a deficiency of this protein fraction might reflect an absence of antibodies, thereby resulting in repeated infections. Simplistic as this concept now sounds, in 1952 Bruton had a difficult time convincing academicians of the significance of his discovery. It remained for his group to devise a trial of gamma globulin therapy for the child. Remarkably, the dosage decided upon was very close to that which would currently be recommended, despite the fact that little was known at that time of metabolism and serum levels of immunoglobulins. A final twist to this story is that the disorder described by Bruton was probably the primary acquired form of hypogammaglobulinemia rather than the congenital form. His patient was relatively well until approximately 3 years of age, at which time the child contracted measles. This was followed some 6 months later by the first of the recurrent bacterial infections. Regardless of the precise form of hypogammaglobulinemia, it was Bruton who established the importance of humoral antibodies as a primary component of host defense mechanisms.

Coincident with Bruton's discovery, case reports appeared in the Swiss and German literature of children with a different type of immune deficiency.[9] Both girls and boys were reported on, and the disease followed a far more fulminant course than that of Bruton's patient. Afflicted children usually developed symptoms within the first month of life, and death was inevitably within the first year or two. Not only were bacterial infections a problem, but viral and fungal pathogens were also involved. Steatorrhea, wasting, and eczematoid rashes were common clinical findings. It was recognized that this disorder, first called "Swiss agammaglobulinemia," involved a combined deficiency of the humoral and cellular immune systems. At about this time, the role of the thymus as a central organ ·in the development of the cell-mediated immune system was appreciated, and it was recognized that children with Swiss agammaglobulinemia lacked a functional thymus. Subsequently, a group of diseases have been recognized within the general category of severe combined immune deficiency (SCID).[10] These disorders, of diverse etiology, have in common combined deficiency of the humoral and cellular immune systems.

The third basic disorder of the immune system was described by a Philadelphia endocrinologist, Dr. Angelo DiGeorge, in 1968.[11] DiGeorge described a patient with a combined defect of hypoparathyroidism and absence of the thymus. Immunologically, the patient had a primary defect of cell-mediated immunity, with relatively little evidence of humoral immune deficiency. As was the case with hypogammaglobulinemia and SCID, the DiGeorge syndrome is now recognized as the prototype of disorders involving structures common to the embryologic sites of the third to fourth branchial arches. A heterogeneous group of disorders, involving combinations of the thyroid and parathyroid glands, thymus, and great vessels has been described, sharing in common a primary defect of cell-mediated immunity with variable involvement of humoral immunity.

It was thus considered that patients with recurrent infections had defects involving either the humoral immune system (prototype: Bruton's disease), the cell-mediated immune system (prototype: DiGeorge syndrome), or a combined deficiency of humoral and cell-mediated immunity (prototype: Swiss agammaglobulinemia). In 1966, however, an entirely new set of parameters was introduced into the clinical spectrum of disorders causing recurrent infections. Holmes and co-workers studied patients with a disorder now known as chronic granulomatous disease (CGD).[12] This disorder, characterized by indolent infections of a granulomatous nature, afflicted males and ended with death, usually by the first decade of life. A primary defect in bactericidal activity of polymorphonuclear leukocytes (PMN) from afflicted boys was observed. PMN from their mothers (obligate carriers in an X-linked disorder) had intermediate bactericidal activity between PMN from patients and from normal controls. Subsequently, Baehner and Nathan demonstrated a primary metabolic aberration in the functionally defective PMN, thereby establishing a biochemical defect as the primary cause of decreased bactericidal activities.[13]

For several reasons, these observations were of major importance. First, they provided the first described inborn error of PMN function. As such, the discovery was of great interest to geneticists, developmental biologists, and a broad base of scientific and clinical subspecialists. The recognition that a metabolic abnormality provided the basis of the functional disorder also spurred intense interest within the biochemical community. Accordingly, a group of disorders are now recognized within the category of CGD, although the precise biochemical lesions remain to be characterized. Second, and more relevant to our purpose, was the recognition that if a deficiency of one function of the PMN—in this case bactericidal activity—could lead to recurrent infections in a patient, then defects in other PMN functions, such as movement or phagocytosis, might also lead to recurrent infections. In the last decade, this hypothesis has proven true, and an entire spectrum of disorders of PMN and, more recently, mononuclear leukocyte (MNL) functions have been recognized. Although comprising a major portion of "new" science in clinical medicine, it should be remembered that the existence of such defects was predicted by the Nobel Prize-winning work of Elie Metchnikoff around the turn of the century.[14] We in clinical medicine are just beginning to catch up with the genius of Metchnikoff.

In parallel with the recognition of a cellular and humoral component to the basic immune response—i.e., the T- and B-cell systems—is the recognition of a number of humoral mediators that interact with the phagocytic systems. Among the best studied of these systems is the serum complement system, a series of proteins that interact in modulating such processes as opsonization and chemotaxis. Clinical abnormalities of the complement system are varied, ranging from hereditary angio-edema to syndromes of severe recurrent infections.[15,16] As we shall see, complement may play an even broader role in host defenses by also modulating components of T- and B-cell activities. Other mediators, such as coagulation-derived factors, may also be important in host defenses, although less is known of their biologic significance.

Any evaluation of the compromised host must, therefore, consider these four major aspects of the immune-inflammatory response: humoral immunity (B-cell system), cell-mediated immunity (T-cell system), phagocytic cell systems (polymorphonuclear leukocytes, monocytes, and macrophages), and humoral mediators or amplifiers, including complement- and coagulation-derived factors. The following chapters review these components as they occur in the fetus and neonate.

REFERENCES

1. McCracken GH Jr, Nelson JD: Antimicrobial Therapy for Newborns. New York, Grune & Stratton, 1977
2. McCracken GH, Shinefield HR: Changes in the pattern of neonatal septicemia and meningitis. Am J Dis Child 112: 33–39, 1966
3. Stagno S, Volanakis J, Reynolds DW, et al: Virus-host interactions in perinatally acquired cytomegalovirus infections of man: Comparative studies on antigenic load and immune complex formation, in Cooper MD, Dayton DH (eds): Development of Host Defenses. New York, Raven Press, 1977, pp 237–250
4. Goldman AS, Smith CW: Host resistance factors in human milk. J Pediatr 82:1082–1090, 1973
5. Pitt J: Breast milk leukocytes. Pediatrics 58:769–770, 1976
6. Beer AE: Immunologic benefits and hazards of milk in the maternal-perinatal relationship, in Moore TD (ed): Necrotizing Enterocolitis in the Newborn Infant, Report of the Sixty-Eighth Ross Conference on Pediatric Research. Columbus, Ohio, Ross Laboratories, 1975
7. Goldblum RM, Ahlstedt S, Carlson B, et al: Antibody production by human colostrum cells, abstracted. Pediatr Res 9:330, 1975
8. Bruton OD: Agammaglobulinemia. Pediatrics 9:722–728, 1952
9. Hitzig WH: Congenital thymic and lymphocytic deficiency disorders, in Stiehm ER, Fulginiti VA (eds): Immunologic Disorders in Infants and Children. Philadelphia, Saunders, 1973
10. Ammann AJ: T cell and T-B cell immunodeficiency disorders. Pediatr Clin North Am 24:293–311, 1977
11. DiGeorge AM: Congenital absence of the thymus and its immunologic consequences: Concurrence with congenital hypoparathyroidism. Birth Defects 4:116, 1968
12. Holmes B, Quie PG, Windhorst DB, et al: Fetal granulomatous disease of childhood: An inborn abnormality of phagocytic function. Lancet i:1225–1228, 1966
13. Baehner RL, Nathan DG: Quantitative nitroblue tetrazolium test in chronic granulomatous disease. N Engl J Med 278:971–976, 1968

14. Metchikoff E: Lectures on the Comparative Pathology of Inflammation. New York, Dover Publications, 1968
15. Johnston RB Jr, Stroud RM: Complement and host defense against infection. J Pediatr 90:169–179, 1977
16. Spitzer RE: The complement system. Pediatr Clin North Am 24:341–364, 1977

2

Development of the T-Cell System

Significant gaps remain in our understanding of the functional status of the T-cell system in neonates. In particular, maturational events leading from a stage of unresponsiveness to the elaboration of specific immunity are poorly characterized. The initial appearance of lymphocytes in fetal tissues occurs at approximately 40 days of gestation.[1] Some controversy has surrounded the origin of these cells. Early work suggested that the lymphocytes differentiated from precursor cells of the thymic rudiment itself, either directly from epithelial cells or from mesenchymal cells that penetrate into the thymic epithelial anlage and there undergo lymphoid differentiation.[2] More recent evidence gathered from two entirely different experimental approaches now suggests, however, that most, if not all, of the lymphocytes appearing in the thymus are derived from blood-borne stem cells.

The first of these approaches utilized sex chromosomes as cell markers. In such studies, Moore and Owen[3] and Owen and Ritter[4] demonstrated migration of cells into the thymus from the circulation.

The second approach utilized a unique cell marking technique[5] based upon structural differences in the nuclear structure of two species of birds closely related in taxonomy, the Japanese quail *(Coturnix coturnix japonica)* and the chick *(Gallus gallus)*. In the quail, the nucleolus is hypertrophied in all adult and embryonic cells owing to the presence of large amounts of heterochromatic DNA. By contrast, chromatin in chick nucleoli is evenly dispersed and contributes little to nucleolar structure. Quail and chick cells, when present in chimeras, can thus be easily distinguished after Feulgen staining. Upon analysis of chick–quail chimeras at various embryonic stages, the following conclusions were drawn:

1. The thymus is made up of cells of several embryonic origins.
2. Medullary and cortical reticular cells originate from the pharyngeal endoderm.
3. The connective cells emanate from the cephalic neural crest and are of mesectodermal origin.
4. The endothelial cells of the blood vessels are of mesodermal origin.
5. The lymphoid population is derived from blood-borne precursor cells and may, therefore, be considered as mesodermal derivatives.

The hematopoietic stem cells from liver, spleen, and perhaps, bone marrow enter the thymus at approximately 8 weeks of gestation,[6] where they are endowed with surface antigens. In the mouse, there are at least three distinct surface markers—Ly 1+, 2+, 3+ phenotype and Ly 2+, 3+ phenotype. These phenotypes appear in the order of Ly 2+, 3+; Ly 1+, 2+, 3+, and finally, well after birth, Ly 1+.[7] Although T-cell antigens in humans analogous to specific T-cell antigens (theta antigen) in mice have not yet been identified, they are presumed to exist.[6]

QUANTITATIVE MEASUREMENTS OF T CELLS

Detection of T cells in fetal and neonatal life is still in a preliminary stage. Wybran and co-workers studied T-cell development in 13 human fetuses, ranging from 11 to 19 months, by the sheep red blood cell rosette technique.[8] The formation of rosettes (E-rosettes) between human lymphocytes and sheep red blood cells is generally regarded as a property of human thymus-derived lymphocytes. In their studies, the thymus contained a maximum of 65 percent rosette-forming cells (RFC). Upon modifying the assay by incubation of the lymphocytes in fetal calf serum, a substantial increase in the percentage of RFC in 12 human fetuses was observed.[9]

Hayward and Ezer found that 50 to 96 percent of thymus lymphocytes formed E-rosettes from 13 fetuses aged 15 to 26 weeks' gestation.[10] Only 0 to 41 percent of spleen cells formed E-rosettes.

A number of investigators have reported decreased numbers of T cells in cord blood. Campbell and co-workers[11] and Smith and co-workers[12] utilized the long incubation E-rosette technique, while Davis and Galant found both the "active" and total rosette-forming cells to be decreased in cord blood.[13] Active rosettes are those rapid rosette formers read following a short incubation.[14] Viral or neoplastic diseases may be associated with decreased numbers of active rosettes. Total rosettes, which are read following a longer incubation period, are thought to reflect total numbers of T cells.[14] Diaz-Jouanen and co-workers also found decreased percentages of T cells in cord blood of newborns when studied by E-rosettes but no signficant decrease when studied by indirect immunofluorescence.[15] The latter technique utilized a rabbit antihuman fetal thymocyte antiserum absorbed with B cells derived from patients with chronic lymphocytic leukemia. In exploration of this discrepancy, the authors suggested that the low E-rosette values were perhaps related to immaturity of small tentaclelike projections and outpouchings on T cells. Using electron microscopy, such outpouchings are more prominent on B than on T cells. Whatever the explanation proves to be, this dichotomy suggests potential heterogeneity among T-cell populations as discriminated by immunofluorescent and rosetting techniques.

A disadvantage of the use of cord blood for such studies is the potential contamination with maternal blood. Several authors have studied T-cell populations in peripheral venous blood of neonates. Christiansen and co-workers evaluated T-cell numbers in 29 healthy neonates and 16 mothers.[16] Percentages of T lymphocytes (E-rosettes) were significantly decreased (p < 0.001). In a similar study, Ferguson and co-workers studied venous blood from 20 Caucasian infants of 28 to 40 weeks' gestation, of whom 10 were small for gestational age (SGA).[17] No significant differences were found between percentages of T lymphocytes in peripheral blood from adults and those from the appropriate for gestational age (AGA) infants. (There is no apparent explanation for the differences in results on AGA babies in these two studies.) A highly provocative finding in the Ferguson study was a significantly decreased pecentage of T cells in blood from SGA babies compared with that from AGA babies. Little is known of immunologic maturation in SGA babies, and collection of such data will likely provide a difficult but valuable quest in the future.

It should be noted that the above studies deal with percentages rather than with total numbers of T cells in cord blood. The latter are generally increased in cord blood owing to the absolute lymphocytosis in the newborn.[11,15]

MEASUREMENTS OF T-CELL FUNCTION
(TABLE 2-1)

Antigen recognition

The initial step in the specific immune response is the recognition of certain antigens as foreign. Among the methods used to measure antigen recognition in vitro is the mixed leukocyte culture (MLC). In this technique, the proliferative response of lymphocytes upon incubation with mitomycin-treated cells of foreign

Table 2-1
T-Cell Functions in the Human Fetus

Function	Fetal Age First Reported	Text Reference
Antigen recognition	12 weeks	24–26
Antigen binding	10 to 13 weeks	27
Cell-mediated lympholysis	7 months (not studied earlier)	28
Antibody-dependent cytotoxicity (may not be T-cell function)	Cord blood (not studied earlier)	11, 41
Graft-versus-host reactivity	13 weeks	35
Mitogenic stimulation	12 to 22 weeks	43, 47–50
Antigenic stimulation	Newborns (not studied earlier	44, 46, 54, 55
Lymphotoxin production	Cord blood (not studied earlier)	56
Interferon production	Indeterminate	57, 58

origin is measured by incorporation of a radiolabeled nucleic acid precursor, such as tritiated thymidine. The MLC presumably represents the recognition phase in the response of T lymphocytes to foreign histocompatibility antigens in vitro.

MLC reactions have been obtained with cells from human fetal thymus, spleen, and liver as responders. Initial studies suggested that the earliest site of immunologically competent responding cells was fetal liver (as early as 10 weeks of gestation), followed by thymic lymphocytes (12 to 16 weeks) and by blood and splenic lymphocytes (16 weeks).[18] The mere presence of a proliferative response in an MLC reaction is not, however, definitive proof of immunologic competence, since even immunologically incompetent cells may respond to blastogenic factors derived from the stimulating T cells.[19-23] Asantila and Toivanen explored this problem using a cell-suicide technique.[24] In this method, fetal cells were first stimulated with a foreign antigen. Cells responding to the antigen were next eliminated with BUDR and ultraviolet light, and the remaining cells were then exposed to a new stimulant. If the initial response was nonspecific, the vast majority of the responding cells were activated by the first stimulant, and little response occurred upon introduction of the second stimulant. If an immunologically specific activation occurred with the first stimulant, however, only that clone of responders was activated, and a new antigenic stimulant could activate a separate specific clone.

Utilizing this technique, Asantila and co-workers showed that proliferative responses of fetal liver cells were immunologically nonspecific and that immunologically specific reactions were obtainable only with thymic and splenic lymphocytes.[25,26] Human fetal thymus lymphocytes could distinguish allogeneic lymphocytes of different origin by 12 weeks' gestation, and splenic lymphocytes acquired this property by 15 weeks' gestation. These findings were recently duplicated in the fetal lamb, where cells capable of specific recognition first appeared in the thymus 58 days after conception and in the spleen at 70 days.[24] When compared with adult sheep peripheral blood lymphocytes, fetal thymus or spleen cells were equally reactive. Fetal lamb lymphocytes were also capable of recognizing intraspecies differences on xenogeneic (mouse, human) cells.

Antigen Binding by Fetal Lymphocytes

Dwyer and co-workers used autoradiography to study antigen binding of ^{125}I-labeled flagellin from *Salmonella adelaide* and hemocyanin from *Jasus lalandii*.[27] Cells from 22 human fetal thymuses, ranging from 10 to 30 weeks' gestation, and thymic biopsies from children and adults obtained at cardiac surgery were studied. The mean number of antigen-binding cells was highest in fetal thymus, 182 per 10^4 lymphocytes compared with 60 per 10^4 lymphocytes in thymuses of children and 5 per 10^4 lymphocytes from adult thymuses. Antigen binding was blocked by preincubation of thymocytes with either anti-μ or anti-light-chain sera.

Cell-mediated Lympholysis

A natural consequence of antigen recognition in immunologically mature hosts is the activation of "effector" cells. Little is known of the development of effector cells during early human ontogeny. Granberg and co-workers[28] studied this problem by cell-mediated lympholysis (CML).[29] In this system, effector lymphocytes are first sensitized by an MLC reaction. Such sensitized effector cells are able to lyse suitably prepared target cells, usually allogeneic lymphocytes. Target cells were prepared from lymphocytes of the same donors as the stimulating cells and third-party cells (HLA-unidentical with the stimulating cells). Following labeling with ^{51}Cr, they were then exposed to the sensitized effector cells, and the amount of target cell lysis was determined by measuring chromium release. In a positive CML reaction, significantly more chromium release occurs from the specific target cells than from the third-party targets. Granberg and co-workers studied cord blood from 17 full-term infants and 1 premature infant (gestational age, 7 months).[28] In 6 out of 18 cases, the neonatal capacity for CML equaled that of adult peripheral blood lymphocytes, while all others showed lower values. CML in the 7-month-old premature was equal to the adult value. The authors suggested that the frequently observed low CML activity of neonates might reflect differences of T-cell frequency rather than deficient CML activity. Regardless, they concluded that their observations "unambiguously indicate that CML capacity develops during the intrauterine life of the human fetus."

These results are comparable to those obtained with a presumably less specific lymphocyte mitogen, phytohemagglutinin (PHA). Carr and co-workers demonstrated PHA-induced cytotoxicity of human lymphocytes from term infants against chicken erythrocytes.[30] Campbell et al. found that PHA-induced cytotoxicity of cord lymphocytes against targets derived from a human liver cell line was substantially less than that of adult peripheral blood lymphocytes.[11]

The suggestion that cytotoxic and mitogenic responses to PHA may be functions of different cell populations, or at least differential rates of maturation, was provided by the data of

Stites and co-workers, who observed PHA-induced cytotoxicity against chicken erythrocytes with lymphocytes from bone marrow, spleen, and blood of 14- to 18-week-old human fetuses.[31] Thymocytes from the same fetuses, however, failed to destroy target cells, even though they showed a blastogenic response to PHA. The authors concluded that PHA-dependent cytotoxicity and DNA synthesis (implied by blastogenic response) were functions of different cell populations.

Further evidence of differential maturation of components of mature T-cell function was provided by the studies of Wu and co-workers[32] in mice and by several groups of workers in fetal sheep. Neonatal mouse spleen cells were reactive in MLC, while CML capacity did not develop until 7 days of age. In fetal sheep, Silverstein and Prendergast[33] and Schinckel and Ferguson[34] did not observe rejection of allogeneic skin grafts until approximately midgestation, while Asantila and Toivanen found that thymocytes of a 58-day-old fetal lamb can distinguish allogeneic and xenogeneic (mouse, human) differences on the stimulating cells.[35]

Interpretation of these data into an orderly sequence of differential function of the human T-cell system is not yet possible. Not only are data from the various functional assays inadequate but also many of the assays involve a number of other functions in addition to those being studied. For example, the ability to reject a skin graft involves intact inflammatory as well as immunologic effectors. As discussed in further detail in Chapter 4, inflammatory function in the neonate and fetus may be limiting in full expression of such phenomena as graft rejection. Niederhuber and co-workers, for example, observed rejection of allogeneic renal transplants in fetal lambs with gestation periods ranging from 70 to 130 days.[36] Similar difficulties of interpretation apply to other available studies of graft rejection in mammalian species. Porter found that foreign spleen cells injected in utero into fetal rabbits resulted in immunologic tolerance prior to day 22 but were rejected if introduced after day 22 of fetal life.[37] Homograft rejection by the fetal monkey occurred as early as day 58 of a 165-day gestational period,[38] while similar function in the rat was deficient even at birth.[38,40]

Antibody-dependent Cytotoxicity

Antibody-dependent cytotoxicity may be mediated by a different, perhaps non-T, cell type than PHA-induced cytotoxicity.[29] In this system, the ability of PHA-induced lymphocytes to kill antibody-coated target cells is measured. Data here are somewhat contradictory. Campbell and co-workers found activity of cord blood lymphocytes to approximate that of adult lymphocytes,[11] while Rachelefsky et al. found that antibody-dependent cytotoxic activity of cord blood lymphocytes was extremely low.[41] No explanation exists for this difference. The only apparent variable between the two studies was the source of target cells.

Graft-Versus-Host Reactivity

Asantila and co-workers studied xenogenic immunologic reactivity of human fetal lymphocytes.[35] Splenic lymphocytes from 13-week-old human fetuses caused a local graft-versus-host (GVH) reaction when implanted under a rat kidney capsule. Lymphocytes from 18- to 23-week-old human fetuses were as reactive in GVH as adult human lymphocytes. Fetal thymus cells were less active than fetal spleen cells.

Response to Nonspecific Stimulation

Phytohemagglutinin (PHA) is a plant lectin that has been used extensively in the evaluation of lymphocyte function. Lymphocyte proliferation following culture with soluble PHA is primarily a T-cell response,[42] while culture with locally concentrated or insolubilized PHA may also stimulate B cells.[42]

A number of investigators have observed greater "spontaneous" transformation of cord blood lymphocytes.[30,43-46] Based upon morphology, the increased "spontaneous" transformation occurs by 33 weeks of gestation.[43] Pegrum and co-workers found increased tritiated thymidine uptake in 22 fetal thymic cultures ranging from 16 to 24 weeks' gestation.[47] Poor, if any, responses were obtained from bone marrow or liver cultures, while fetal spleen cultures gave erratic responses. Kay and co-workers demonstrated PHA responsiveness of fetal thymocytes by 17 weeks of gestation.[48] PHA-responsive cells with 46, XY karyotype (presumably of fetal origin) were identified in the maternal circulation at 14 weeks of gestation.[48] Papiernick studied PHA responsiveness of thymocytes from fetuses aged 12 to 22 weeks.[49] Lymphocyte transformation increased progressively until 18 weeks, when the level declined to that of adult thymic lymphocytes. August and co-workers found PHA-responsive lymphocytes in human fetal thymus by 12 weeks of gestation and in spleens 2 to 4 weeks later.[50] In spleens, establishment of the PHA response was associated with the appearance of small lymphocytes in cuffs surrounding central arterioles. Jones[43] and Lindahl-Kiessling and Book[51] found PHA-responsive lymphocytes in 15- to 17-week-old fetuses.

Utilizing time-dose kinetics, Stites and co-workers found PHA responsiveness in human fetuses first in thymus at 10 weeks and then in peripheral blood and spleen 3 to 4 weeks later.[31] Marrow and hepatic lymphoid cells did not respond to this antigen.

PHA responsiveness of cord blood lymphocytes has been found to be greater,[11,31,52] equal to,[11,43,44] and less than[43,53] that of adult lymphocytes.

Alford and co-workers have recently studied this response in detail, utilizing PHA in a concentration that maximally stimulated adult lymphocytes cultured in 20 percent serum.[46] Thymidine uptakes of cord lymphocytes and normal infants less than 20 months old were measured under four different conditions—unstimulated, PHA stimulated, streptokinase-streptodormase (SK-SD) stimulated, and *Candida* extract stimulated. Un-stimulated and PHA-stimulated thymidine uptakes were greater than in adult lymphocytes but gradually decreased to adult values. Specific lymphocyte reactivity to SK-SD was quite low in all groups of infants, while *Candida*-induced transformation was comparable to adult values.

Response to Antigenic Stimulation

This has been less extensively studied than mitogen-induced blastogenesis. Leiken and co-workers demonstrated specific blastogenic response to *Salmonella* antigen by lymphocytes of newborn infants who had been immunized 2 weeks earlier with typhoid vaccine.[54]

Some question exists on the specificity of such transformation. Leiken and Oppenheim found no transformation of lymphocytes from unimmunized neonates when cultured with tetanus and diphtheria toxoids,[44] thereby supporting specificity of neonatal lymphocyte transformation. By contrast, however, Leiken et al. reported significant transformation of cord blood lymphocytes to type I pneumococcus extract and streptolysin O,[55] antigens to which neonates would not likely be exposed.

As cited in the previous section, Alford and co-workers demonstrated blastogenesis toward *Candida* extract in approximately half of the 2-week-old infants tested.[46] Specific reactivity to SK-SD was, by contrast, seldom seen.

Lymphokine Production

LYMPHOTOXIN

Lymphotoxin is a lymphokine that is cytotoxic for a variety of target cells and is produced by lymphocytes exposed to PHA, concanavallin A, a variety of antigens, and allogeneic cells.[56] Eife and co-workers studied lymphotoxin production by cord blood lymphocytes from 17 normal newborn infants and peripheral blood lymphocytes from 12 normal adults. Lymphotoxin production by the newborns was only 40 percent of the value for the adult controls. When a lymphotoxin index (ratio of lymphotoxin production to transformation) was calculated, it was found that, regardless of degree of transformation, newborn lymphocytes only produced approximately 25 percent as much lymphotoxin as did adult lymphocytes.[52]

INTERFERON

Overall and Glascow studied interferon production in fetal lambs.[57] Levels of interferon production in second-and third-trimester lambs were significantly higher than those found in adult sheep. Significantly lower levels were found in animals stimulated during the first trimester. A possibly crucial variable in these studies was the route of inoculation. First-trimester animals were injected intraperitoneally, while second- and third-trimester animals were injected intravenously.

Ray found production of interferon by lymphocytes from human fetuses, cord blood, and term neonates to be equivalent to adult levels.[58]

Little data exist on the relative production of other lymphokines by neonatal lymphocytes.

T-CELL FUNCTION—INDIRECT EVIDENCE

A number of studies indirectly support the development of significant T-cell function during intrauterine life. Maternal leukocytes including immunocompetent lymphocytes may gain access to the fetal circulation.[59,60] If such cells remain viable and proliferate, they might be expected to mount a graft-versus-host (GVH) reaction. This does not occur, however, during normal gestation, which indirectly suggests early acquisition of cellular immunity by the fetus with the consequent ability to reject or inactivate the maternal lymphocytes. In the immunologically incompetent fetus, however, such maternal lymphocytes may cause GVH reactions. Such an instance was reported by Kadowacki and co-workers, who observed a male child with thymic dysplasia and XX/XY chimerism in his circulating lymphocyte population who succumbed to an illness highly reminiscent of GVH disease.[61] This suggests that maternal lymphocytes colonized the fetus and triggered the GVH reaction. Further evidence of probable development of an intact cell-mediated immune response during fetal life is the rarity of GVH reactions documented in fetuses receiving intrauterine transfusions for severe Rh incompatibility.

Only one such case has been even tentatively described,[62] suggesting that the human fetus has generally developed a degree of cellular immunity by 27 weeks, the time that intrauterine transfusions are usually performed.

Yakovac had the rare opportunity to study the thymus of a 14-week-old male embryo whose previous two male siblings had died from severe combined immunodeficiency disease.[63] This fetal thymus, when compared with thymuses from immunologically normal fetuses of similar gestational age, already showed classic histologic findings of combined immunodeficiency. Extrapolation of these data would thus suggest that the normal human fetus develops a partially functional T-cell system by the first trimester.

A number of other poorly characterized examples of possible GVH reactions in immunologically incompetent fetuses have been suggested.[64]

REFERENCES

1. Solomon GB: Lymphopoiesis, in Foetal and Neonatal Immunology. Amsterdam, North Holland, 1971, p 22
2. Metcalf D, Moore MAS: Haemopoietic Cells. Amsterdam, North Holland, 1971
3. Moore MAS, Owen JJT: Experimental studies on the development of the thymus. J Exp Med 129:431–437, 1969
4. Owen JJT, Ritter MA: Tissue interaction in the development of thymus lymphocytes. J Exp Med 129:431–437, 1969
5. Le Douarin N: Thymus ontogeny studied in interspecific chimeras, in Dayton DH, Cooper MD (eds): Development of Host Defenses. New York, Raven Press, 1977
6. Owen JJT, Raff MC: Studies on the differentiation of thymus-derived lymphocytes. J Exp Med 132:1216–1232, 1970
7. Mosier DE, Johnson BM: Ontogeny of mouse lymphocyte function. II. Development of the ability to produce antibody is modulated by T lymphocytes. J Exp Med 141:216–226, 1975
8. Wybran J, Carr MC, Fudenberg HH: The human rosette-forming cells as a marker of a population of thymus-derived cells. J Clin Invest 51:2537–2543, 1972

9. Wybran J, Carr MC, Fudenberg HH: Effect of serum on human rosette-forming cells in fetuses and adult blood. Clin Immunol Immunopathol 1:408–413, 1973

10. Hayward AR, Ezer G: Development of lymphocyte populations in the human foetal thymus and spleen. Clin Exp Immunol 17:169–178, 1974

11. Campbell AC, Waller C, Wood J, et al: Lymphocyte subpopulations in the blood of newborn infants. Clin Exp Immunol 18:469–482, 1974

12. Smith MA, Evans J, Steel CM: Age-related variations in proportion of circulating T cells. Lancet ii:922–924, 1974

13. Davis RH, Galant SP: Nonimmune rosette formation: A measure of the newborn infant's cellular immune response. J Pediatr 87:449–452, 1975

14. Wybran J, Leven AS, Spitler LE, et al: Rosette-forming cells, immunologic deficiency diseases and transfer factor. N Engl J Med 288:710–713, 1973

15. Diaz-Jouanen E, Struckland RG, Williams RC Jr: Studies of human lymphocytes in the newborn and the aged. Am J Med 58:620–628, 1975

16. Christiansen JS, Osther K, Pietersen B, et al: B, T, and null lymphocytes in newborn infants and their mothers. Acta Paediatr Scand 65:425–428, 1976

17. Ferguson AC, Lawlor GJ, Neumann CC, et al: Decreased rosette-forming lymphocytes in malnutrition and intrauterine growth retardation. J Pediatr 85:717–723, 1974

18. Stites DP, Carr MC, Fudenberg HH: Ontogeny of cellular immunity in the human fetus. Development of responses to phytohemagglutinin and to allogeneic cells. Cell Immunol 11:257–271, 1974

19. Kasakura S: A blastogenic factor in unidirectional mixed cultures with x-irradiated cells. Transplantation 11:117–121, 1971

20. Lafferty KJ, Cunningham AJ: A new analysis of allogeneic interactions. Aust J Exp Biol Med Sci 53:27–42, 1975

21. v. Boehmer H: Separation of T and B lymphocytes and their role in the mixed lymphocyte culture. J Immunol 112:70–78, 1974

22. Harrison MR, Paul WE: Stimulus-response in the mixed lymphocyte reaction. J Exp Med 138:1602–1607, 1973

23. Janis M, Bach FH: Potentiation of in vitro lymphocyte reactivity. Nature 225:238–239, 1970

24. Asantila T, Toivanen P: Specificity of allogeneic and xenogeneic cell recognition in the fetal lamb. J Immunol 117:555–561, 1976

25. Asantila T, Vahala J, Toivanen P: Generation of functional diversity of T cell receptors. Immunogenetics 1:407–415, 1974

26. Asantila T, Vahala J, Toivanen P: Response of human fetal lymphocytes in xenogeneic mixed leukocyte culture. Phylogenetic and ontogenetic aspects. Immunogenetics 1:272–290, 1974

27. Dwyer JM, Warner NL, McKay IR: Specificity and nature of the antigen-combining sites on fetal and mature thymus lymphocytes. J Immunol 108:1439–1446, 1972

28. Granberg C, Manninen K, Toivanen P: Cell-mediated lympholysis by human neonatal lymphocytes. Clin Immunol Immunopathol 6:256–263, 1976

29. Holm G, Granksson C, Campbell AC, et al: The cytotoxic activity of lymphocytes from human lymph in vitro. Clin Exp Immunol 17:361–369, 1974

30. Carr MC, Sites DP, Fudenberg HH: Dissociation of responses to phytohemagglutinin and adult allogenic lymphocytes in human foetal lymphoid tissues. Nature (New Biol) 241:279–281, 1973

31. Stites DP, Caldwell J, Carr MC, et al: Ontogeny of immunity in humans. Clin Immunol Immunopathol 4:519–527, 1975

32. Wu LYF, Blanco A, Cooper MD, et al: Ontogeny of B-lymphocytes differentiation induced by pokeweed mitogens. Clin Immunol Immunopathol 5:208–217, 1976

33. Silverstein AM, Prendergast RA: Fetal response to antigenic stimulus. IV. Rejection of skin homografts by the fetal lamb. J Exp Med 119:955–964, 1974

34. Schinckel PG, Ferguson KA: Skin transplantation in the foetal lamb. Aust J Biol Sci 6:533–546, 1953

35. Asantila T, Sorvari T, Hirvonen T, et al: Xenogeneic reactivity of human fetal lymphocytes. J Immunol 111:984–987, 1973

36. Niederhuber JE, Shermeta D, Turcotte JG, et al: Kidney transplantation in the fetal lamb. Transplantation 12:161–166, 1971

37. Porter KA: Runt disease and tolerance in rabbits. Nature (London) 185:789–790, 1960

38. Sterzl J, Silverstein AM: Developmental aspects of immunity. Adv Immunol 6:337–459, 1967

39. Rawles ME: Pigmentation in autoplastic and homoplastic grafts of skin from fetal and newborn hooded rats. Am J Anat 97:79–127, 1955

40. Medawar PB and Woodruff MFA: The induction of tolerance by skin homografts on newborn rats. Immunology 1:27–35, 1958

41. Rachelefsky GS, McConnachie PR, Teresaki PI, et al: Deficient killer function in newborn and young infant lymphocytes, abstracted. Pediatr Res 7:371, 1973

42. Greaves MF, Bauminger L: Activation of T and B lymphocytes by insoluble phytomitogens. Nature (New Biol) 235:67–70, 1972

43. Jones WR: In vitro transformation of fetal lymphocytes. Am J Obstet Gynecol 104:586–592, 1969

44. Leiken S, Oppenheim JJ: Differences in transformation of adult and newborn lymphocytes stimulated by antigen, antibody and antigen-antibody complexes. Cell Immunol 1:468–475, 1970

45. Pulvertaft RJV, Pulvertaft I: Spontaneous "transformation" of lymphocytes from the umbilical and vein. Lancet ii:892–893, 1966

46. Alford RH, Cartwright BB, Sell SH: Ontogeny of human cell-mediated immunity: Age-related variation of in vitro infantile lymphocyte transformation. Infect Immunol 13:1170–1175, 1976

47. Pegrum GD, Ready D, Thompson E: The effect of phytohaemagglutinin on human foetal cells grown in culture. Br J Haematol 15:371–376, 1968

48. Kay HEM, Wolfendale MM, Playfair JHL: Thymocytes and phytohaemagglutinin. Lancet ii:804, 1966

49. Papiernick M: Correlation of lymphocyte transformation and morphology in the human fetal thymus. Blood 36:470–479, 1970

50. August CS, Berkel AE, Discoll S, et al: Onset of lymphocyte function in the developing human fetus. Pediatr Res 5:539–547, 1971

51. Lindahl-Kiessling K, Book JA: Effects of phytomaemagglutinin on leucocytes. Lancet ii:591, 1964

52. Eife RF, Eife G, August CS: Lymphotoxin production and blast cell transformation by cord blood lymphocytes: Dissociated lymphocyte function in newborn infants. Cell Immunol 14:435–442, 1974

53. Ayoub J, Kasakura S: In vitro response of foetal lymphocytes to PHA, and a plasma factor which suppresses the PHA response of adult lymphocytes. Clin Exp Immunol 8:427–434, 1971

54. Leiken S, Mochir-Fatemi F, Park K: Blast transformation of lymphocytes from newborn human infants. J Pediatr 72:510–517, 1968

55. Leiken S. Whang-Peng J, Oppenheim JJ: In vitro transformation of human cord blood lymphocytes by antigens, in Harris J (ed): Proceedings of the Fifth Leukocyte Culture Conference. New York, Academic Press, 1970

56. Eife RF, August CS: Detection of lymphotoxin produced in mixed lymphocyte cultures (MLC): Variation in target cell sensitivity. Cell Immunol 9:163–168, 1973

57. Overall JC Jr, Glasgow LA: Host resistance to virus infection in the fetus: I. Interferon (IF) production, abstracted. Soc Pediatr Res, 1971, p 81

58. Ray CG: The ontogeny of interferon production by human leukocytes. J Pediatr 76:94–98, 1970

59. Desai RG, Creger WF: Maternofetal passage of leukocytes and platelets in man. Blood 21:665–673, 1963
60. Walknowska J, Conte F, Grumbach MM: Practical and theoretical implications of fetal/maternal lymphocyte transfer. Lancet i:1119–1122, 1969
61. Kadowaki J, Zuelzer WW, Brogh AJ, et al: XX/XY lymphoid chimaerism in congenital immunological deficiency syndrome with thymic alymphoplasia. Lancet ii:1152–1155, 1976
62. Naiman JL, Punnett HH, Lischner HW, et al: Possible graft-versus-host reaction after intrauterine transfusion for Rh erythroblastosis fetalis. N Engl J Med 281:697–701, 1969

3
Development of the B-Cell System

B-CELL ONTOGENY

Understanding of the ontogeny of the B-cell system has been aided by the discovery that precursors of plasma cells can be identified through the presence of membrane-associated immunoglobulins. Consequently, the development of highly specific antisera against the various immunoglobulin classes has made it possible to initiate studies of B-cell development.

Two stages of B-cell maturation have been recognized.[1] Raff and co-workers studied the development of the murine B-cell system.[2] In mouse fetal liver and spleen, they observed large lymphoid cells containing intracellular (cytoplasmic) IgM but lacking detectable surface immunoglobulins. These "pre-B" cells were seen in the liver of 12-day-old embryos, while cells demonstrating surface immunoglobulins were not detected until day 17. Pre-B cells were found in bone marrow but not in spleen and lymph nodes.

Gathings and co-workers studied B-cell ontogeny in human abortuses ranging from 7.5 to 16.5 weeks' gestation.[3] Approximately 0.1 percent of liver cells from a 7.5-week-old fetus showed intracellular IgM, while no surface Ig cells of any class were detected. In fetuses ranging from 9.5 to 12.5 weeks' gestational age, liver contained both cytoplasmic-positive and cytoplasmic-surface-positive cells in a ratio of approximately 2:1. Typical mature B lymphocytes were identified in 13- to 16.5-week-old fetuses. IgM was the only intracellular immunoglobulin class detected in any fetus.

Bone marrow from each of 6 fetuses (aged 13 to 16.5 weeks) examined contained pre-B cells. None, however, were found in spleen or peripheral blood even when secretory IgM lymphocytes constituted 10 to 40 percent of mononuclear cells.

These pre-B cells are probably comparable to B lymphocyte precursors described by other workers. Ryser and Vassalli[4] and Osmond and Nossal[5] described populations of marrow lymphocytes capable of rapid differentiation from negative-surface immunoglobulin to positive-surface immunoglobulin. Melchers and co-workers demonstrated large immunoglobulin-synthesizing lymphoid cells in 10- to 12-day-old mouse embryos and in 13- to 15-day-old fetal liver.[6] Small immunoglobulin-synthesizing lymphocytes occurred at 15 to 16 days, which correlates with the time at which surface-bearing immunoglobulin cells can be demonstrated.

ONTOGENY OF IMMUNOGLOBULIN
CLASS-SPECIFIC B CELLS

Another aspect of B-cell development that has been studied through these techniques is the order of expression of individual immunoglobulin classes on B-cell surfaces. Lawton and co-workers first detected surface IgM-positive cells in liver of fetuses aged 9.5 to 10 weeks.[7] Cells bearing surface IgD were not found until 12 weeks of age. Surface IgG-bearing cells were found in 3 of 5 fetuses aged 9.5 to 10 weeks, while surface IgA-positive cells were identified at about the same time as IgD. This, and other data,[8-10] suggested that B lymphocytes emerged sequentially in a specific chronology of embryogenesis by an antigen-independent process. The order of development of the immunoglobulin classes was IgM, IgG, and IgA. Expression of IgD followed IgM and did not clearly precede IgG or IgA.

A prevailing question concerns the anatomic site in mammals responsible for the induction of primary B-cell development. Although the question has not been definitively answered, Lawton and Cooper have summarized data suggesting that fetal liver and adult bone marrow normally serve sequentially as the mammalian bursa equivalent[1] (Table 3-1).

Table 3-1

Characteristics of B Cells in Fetal Liver and Adult Bone Marrow, Suggesting That These Organs Serve as Bursa-Equivalent Sites

	Fetal Liver	Bone Marrow
Site at which B cells are first detectable	+	
Presence of pre-B cells in the fetus and adult	+	+
De novo generation of B lymphocytes in organ culture*	+	+
High ratio of sIgM$^+$ sIgD$^-$ to sIgM$^+$ sIgD$^+$ B lymphocytes	+	+
Presence of easily tolerizable (immature) B lymphocytes	+	+

*Fetal spleen shares this property. Since pre-B cells are present in fetal liver by 12 days' gestation in the mouse, it is possible that traffic of pre-B cells to spleen and bone marrow may explain de novo development of B lymphocytes in either or both organs.

From Lawton AR, Cooper MD: Two new stages of antigen-independent B cell development in mice and humans, in Cooper MD, Dayton DH (eds): Development of Host Defenses. New York, Raven Press, 1977, pp 43–54.

ANTIGEN-DEPENDENT B-CELL DIFFERENTIATION

The second stage of B-cell differentiation is antigen dependent. This may result from exposure of B cells either to specific antigens or to nonspecific lectins such as pokeweed mitogen. In 15-week-old human fetuses, splenic and blood B lymphocytes were triggered to differentiate into IgG- or IgA-producing plasma cells by stimulation with pokeweed mitogen. IgG and IgA responses remained less than that of IgM, however, until 2 to 3 months postnatally.[11] This difference might be explained by developmental T-cell function, since the B-cell response to pokeweed in humans is T-cell dependent.[12]

The same considerations hold for antigens, the majority of which are thymus dependent and require both specific and nonspecific factors for activation. Differentiation of pure B-cell populations into immunoglobulin-secreting cells occurs infrequently, if at all.[13] Isolated populations of suppressor T cells can inhibit antibody production by normally reactive B cells.[14-16] T cells may regulate B-cell functions through direct contact or through the elaboration of factors that may be either cooperative—i.e., amplify B-cell output[17,18]—or suppressive—i.e., inhibit B-cell differentiation[19]—perhaps by induction of a reversible loss of immunoglobulins from the surface of B cells. Modulation of B-cell responses by T cells is significant, and a better understanding of the nature of such interactions will be necessary before full characterization of the neonatal B-cell response will be possible.

ANTIGEN EXPOSURE

The quantitative results of antigen-dependent B-cell differentiation are obviously influenced by the amount of antigen exposure occurring during fetal life. Under lack of such stimulation, lymphoid tissues in mammalian fetuses mature slowly.[20] Thorbecke (21) showed that animals raised from birth in a germfree environment have delayed development of lymphoid organs.[21]

Maternal Transfer

Immune responsiveness may be influenced by fetal sensitization to antigens to which the mother has been exposed.[22-29] In fetal lambs, anti-*Salmonella* bactericidal activity was found in sera of fetuses of more than 75 days' gestation.[20] The antibody was of high molecular weight, 2-mercaptoethanol sensitive, and presumably represented IgM of fetal origin. It was suggested that the lamb was sensitized by antigen absorbed from the maternal gut.

Gill and co-workers studied three aspects of the maternal–fetal immunologic interaction in genetically inbred rats and in man:[28] (1) An aggregated synthetic polypeptide was used to immunize female rats prior to mating, Immunologic capabilities of the offspring were affected by maternal immunization. The effect depended upon the genotype of the strain. The immune responses in the offspring were affected by maternal immunization. The effect depended upon the genotype of the strain. The immune response in the offspring of genetically low responders could be increased and that of high responders decreased by maternal immunization. (2) Lymphocyte reactivity to a panel of five antigens was studied in 48 human maternal–fetal pairs. On occasion, cord blood lymphocytes of fetal origin were reactive to antigens that failed to elicit a response from corresponding maternal lymphocytes. It was suggested that the fetal cells were stimulated by the transplacental passage of antigen. Comparative studies in autologous and in normal AB plasma showed that there were no factors in either the maternal or the fetal circulation at the time of delivery that might have altered the immunologic reactivity of the lymphocytes. (3) Production of migration-inhibiting factor (MIF) was studied during heterozygous and homozygous pregnancies in inbred rats. Inbred animals produced MIF only during heterozygous pregnancies, and the levels increased progressively to delivery and then precipitously declined, suggesting that the interaction of mother and fetus elicits a substantial immune response in heterozygous pregnancies.

A number of other studies have also implicated a role for maternally transmitted antigens in the expression of the fetal–neonatal antibody response.[30-33] Positive skin test reactions have been observed in newborns against common allergens[31] and tuberculoprotein[32,33] presumably transferred to the fetus across the placental barrier.

Amniotic Fluid Transfer

Another source of antigen exposure to the fetus may be through the amniotic fluid. Richardson and Conner injected *Brucella* antigen into the amniotic fluid of fetal lambs.[34] When introduced in late pregnancy, offspring demonstrated both primary and secondary immune responses to *Brucella* antigen. Where twin fetuses were present in separate amniotic fluid sacs, only the fetus sensitized by amniotic fluid injection (subsequently ingested) developed antibody.

Intrauterine Infections

When stimulated with excess antigen in utero, as for example, following intrauterine infections, the human fetus exhibits increased B-cell activity through elevated levels of IgM.[35-37]

Quantitative measurements of B cells in neonatal cord blood have been undertaken primarily with the technique of surface immunofluorescence. In available studies, numbers of B cells and nonreactive "null" cells were increased in cord blood owing to the absolute lymphocytosis in the newborn.[38,39]

FETAL IMMUNOGLOBULIN PRODUCTION

Quantitative Aspects

Several studies utilizing incorporation of radiolabeled amino acids into immunoglobulin have demonstrated synthesis of immunoglobulins during early fetal life. Gitlin and Biasucci found IgM synthesis by 10.5 weeks in human fetal tissue, followed by IgG synthesis at 12 weeks and IgA at 30 weeks.[40] Van Furth and co-workers[41] found immunoglobulin production after the 20th week of gestation and subsequently confirmed these findings with immunofluorescent techniques.[42]

IgG

Fetal synthesis of IgG is minimal.[43] Passively transferred IgG from the maternal circulation occurs as early as day 38.[44] The level remains fairly constant until the 17th week, at which time a proportionate increase occurs with gestational age. At term, cord IgG levels are 5 to 10 percent greater than corresponding maternal levels.[45] Gitlin has proposed a dual mechanism of transfer of IgG—passive and active—to explain the relatively normal IgG levels found in most infants regardless of whether maternal concentrations are increased or decreased.

IgG levels in the premature infant may be proportionately decreased with degree of prematurity.[46-49] Small for gestational age (SGA) babies have even lower levels which may reflect placental dysfunction.[49,50] The significance of this data is unclear, as gamma globulin injections have not conclusively decreased frequency of infections in such infants.[51,52]

IgA

IgA is first detected in human fetuses at 30 weeks of gestation.[53] Synthesis is usually limited until after birth, so that levels seldom exceed 5 mg/dl. Little, if any, IgA is transferred across the placenta.[43]

IgM

From a clinical and functional point of view, IgM synthesis in the human fetus has been of particular interest. Since IgM is not transferred across the placenta in appreciable amounts, that found in cord or neonatal blood is assumed to be of fetal origin. Confirmation of this assumption has been provided by analysis of genetic markers of paternal nature present at birth.[54-56] An elevated cord IgM level suggests the possibility of a congenital infection.[35-37, 57-59] Since this response is caused by exposure to antigens, it is imprecise and subject to the same general variables that influence antibody responses. These include the type of infections, the length of antigen exposure, and the maturity of the fetus when exposed. An elevated IgM level is not diagnostic of a specific infection. Such a diagnosis requires demonstration of either specific antibody titers or reactions with a given test antigen by immunofluorescence.[43]

Specific Antibody Production

Understanding of the fetal antibody response was given impetus by the classic studies of Silverstein in the fetal lamb.[20] A model was developed where indwelling catheters were placed in the cervical vessels of fetal lambs, thus allowing injection of antigens into the fetal circulation and withdrawal of blood samples without surgical intervention. Those studies revealed two major aspects of the fetal antibody response. First, it was clearly shown that fetal lambs were able to produce antibodies in response to antigenic stimulation. Second, was the highly provocative observation that a "hierarchy" of antigen responsiveness existed. In other words, the fetal lamb developed the ability to respond to different antigens at varying periods of fetal life. While antibodies against bacteriophage ϕX 174 were elicited by days 35 to 41 of gestation, ferritin response did not occur until day 66 nor egg albumin response until day 125 of gestation. At term (150 days' gestation), fetal lambs still did not respond to *Salmonella* antigen. A similar stepwise maturation of antibody response has been demonstrated in the opposum[60] and in the rat.[61]

Two basic explanations may be considered in explaining this antigen hierarchy. First, one might hypothesize the emergence of clones of antibody-producing cells in a chronology similar to that seen following administration of the various antigens. Although this is not ruled out, no published data support this explanation.

Alternatively, the hierarchy might involve afferent mechanisms of the immune response, such as the ability to catabolize or process antigens into appropriate instructional materials for T- and/or B-cell activation. There are some data in support of this hypothesis. In C57B1 mice, Braun and Lasky were able to increase the antibody response to sheep erythrocytes in 2-day-old animals by the addition of adult macrophages.[62] Argyris obtained similar results with C3H/He mice.[63]

In a more extensive set of experiments, Blaese studied the role of macrophages in the antibody response in fetal rats.[64] Two antigens were selected against which the newborn rat does not produce antibodies—sheep red blood cells (SRBC) and burro red blood cells (BRBC). When oil-induced peritoneal macrophages from adult rats were administered along with SRBC or BRBC, newborn rats showed excellent antibody responses. Adult rat lymphocytes did not appear to enhance the neonatal antibody response, since lymphocyte-free peritoneal exudate preparations were effective, while spleen cells from adult rats equal in number to the total number of cells in the peritoneal exudate preparations were ineffective. In irradiated animals, peritoneal macrophages were unable to promote antibody responses.

REFERENCES

1. Lawton AR, Cooper MD: Two new stages of antigen-independent B cell development in mice and humans, in Cooper MD, Dayton DH (eds): Development of Host Defenses. New York, Raven Press, 1977, p 43

2. Raff MC, Jegson M, Owen JJT, et al: Early production of intracellular IgM by B-lymphocyte precursors in mouse. Nature 259:224–226, 1976

3. Gathings WE, Cooper MD, Lawton AR, et al: B cell ontogeny in humans, abstracted. Fed Proc 35:276, 1976

4. Ryser J-E, Vassalli P: Mouse bone marrow lymphocytes and their differentiation. J Immunol 113:719–728, 1974

5. Osmond DG, Nossal GJV: Differentiation of lymphocytes in mouse bone marrow. II. Kinetics of maturation and renewal of antiglobulin-binding cells studied by double labeling. Cell Immunol 13:132–145, 1974

6. Melchers F, Von Boehmer H, Phillips RA: B-lymphocyte subpopulations in the mouse. Transplant Rev 25:26–58, 1975

7. Lawton AR, Self KS, Royal SA, et al: Ontogeny of B-lymphocytes in the human fetus. Clin Immunol Immunopathol 1:84–93, 1972

8. Gupta S, Pahwa R, O'Reilly RO, et al: Ontogeny of lymphocyte subpopulations in human fetal liver. Proc Natl Acad Sci USA 73:919–922, 1976

9. Hayward AR, Ezer G: Development of lymphocyte populations in the human foetal thymus and spleen. Clin Exp Immunol 17:169–178, 1974

10. Vossen MJJ: The development of the B immune system in man. Doctoral thesis, University of Leiden, The Neitherlands, Bronder-Offset BV, Rotterdam, 1975

11. Wu LYF, Blanco A, Cooper Md, et al: Ontogeny of B-lymphocyte differentiation induced by pokeweed mitogen. Clin Immunol Immunopathol 5:208–217, 1976

12. Cooper MD, Keightley RG, Lawton AR: Defective T and B cells in primary immunodeficiencies, in Seligmann M, Preud'homme JL, Kourilsky FM (eds): Membrane Receptors of Lymphocytes. Amsterdam, North Holland, 1975, p 431

13. Janossy G, Greaves M: Functional analysis of murine and human B-lymphocyte subsets. Transplant Rev 24:177–236, 1975

14. Gershon RK: T cell control of antibody production. Contemp Top Immunobiol 3:1–40, 1974

15. Tse H, Dutton RW: Separation of helper and suppressor T lymphocytes on a Ficol velocity sedimentation gradient. J Exp Med 143:1119–1210, 1976

16. Waldman TA, Broder S, Blaese RM, et al: Role of suppressor T cells in the pathogeneis of common variable hypogammaglobulinemia. Lancet ii:609–613, 1974

17. Schimpl A, Wecker E: Replacement of T cell function by a T-cell product. Nature (New Biol) 237:15–17, 1972

18. Feldman M, Basten A: Specific collaboration between T and B lymphocytes across a cell impermeable membrane in vitro. Nature (New Biol) 237:13–15, 1972

19. Rich RR, Pierce CW: Biological expression of lymphocyte activation. III. Suppression of plaque-forming cell responses in vitro by supernatant fluid from Con A-activated spleen cell cultures. J Immunol 112:1360–1368, 1974

20. Sterzl J, Silverstein AM: Developmental aspects of immunity. Adv Immunol 6:337–459, 1967

21. Thorbecke GJ: Some histological and functional aspects of lymphoid tissue in germfree animals. I. Morphological studies. Ann NY Acad Sci 78:237–246, 1959

22. Uphoff DE: Maternal control of the immune response. Transplant Proc 5:197–199, 1973

23. Auerbach R, Clark S: Immunological tolerance: Transmission from mother to offspring. Science 189:811–813, 1975

24. Shinka S, Dohi Y, Komatsu T, et al: Immunological unresponsiveness in mice. I. Immunological unresponsiveness induced in embryonic mice by maternofetal transfer of human α-globulin. Biken J 17:59–72, 1974

25. Kindred B, Roelants GE: Restricted clonal response to DNP in adult offspring of immunized mice: A maternal effect. J Immunol 113:445–448, 1974

26. Davis BK, Gill TJ III: Decreased anitbody response in the offspring of immunized high responder rats. J Immunol 115:1166–1168, 1974

27. Gill TJ III, Kunz HW, Bernard CF: Maternal–fetal interaction and immunological memory. Science 172:1346–1348, 1971
28. Gill TJ III, Rabin BS, Kunz HW, et al: Immunologic aspects of maternal-fetal interactions, in Dayton DH, Cooper MD (eds): The Development of Host Defenses. New York, Raven Press, 1977, p 287
29. Adler FL, Noelle RJ: Enduring antibody responses in "normal" rabbits to maternal immunoglobulin allotypes. J Immunol 115:620–625, 1975
30. Leiken S, Oppenheim JJ: Differences in transformation of adult and newborn lymphocytes stimulated by antigen, antibody and antigen–antibody complexes. Cell Immunol 1:468–475, 1970
31. Hashem N: Is maternal lymphocyte sensitization passed to the child? Lancet i:40–41, 1972
32. Stastny P: Accelerated graft rejection in the offspring of immunized mothers. J Immunol 95:929–936, 1965
33. Kruger G, Stolpmann HS: Postnatal development of lymph nodes in mice after prenatal antigenic stimulation. Z Immunitaetsforsch 142:115–121, 1971
34. Richardson M, Conner GH: Prenatal immunization by the oral route: Stimulation of *Brucella* antibody in fetal lambs. Infect Immun 5:454–460, 1972
35. Alford CA: Immunologic status of the newborn. Hosp Practice 5:88–94, 1970
36. Sever JL, White LR: Intrauterine viral infections. Annu Rev Med 19:471–486, 1968
37. Stiehm ER, Ammann AJ, Cherry J: Elevated cord macroglobulins in the diagnosis of intrauterine infections. N Engl J Med 275:971–977, 1966
38. Campbell AC, Waller C, Wood J, et al: Lymphocyte subpopulations in the blood of newborn infants. Clin Exp Immunol 18:469–482, 1974
39. Diaz-Jouanen E, Struckland RG, Williams RC Jr: Studies of human lymphocytes in the newborn and the aged. Am J Med 58:620–628, 1975
40. Gitlin D, Biasucci A: Development of gamma-G, gamma-A, gamma-M, beta IC/beta 1A, Cl esterase inhibitor, ceruloplasmin, transferrin, hemopexin, haptoglobin, fibrinogen, plasminogen, alpha 1-antitrypsin, orosomucoid, beta-lipoprotein, alpha 2-macroglobulin, and prealbumin in the human conceptus. J Clin Invest 48:1422–1446, 1969
41. Van Furth R, Schuit HRE, Hijmans W: The immunological development of the human fetus. J Exp Med 122:1173–1188, 1965
42. Van Furth R, Schuit HRE, Hijmans W: The formation of immuno-

globulins by human tissues in vitro. I. The methods and their specificity. Immunology 11:1–12, 1966

43. Miller ME, Stiehm ER: Phagocytic, opsonic and immunoglobulin studies in newborns. Calif Med 119:43–63, 1973

44. Gitlin D: Development and metabolism of the immune globulins, in Kagen, B, Stiehm, ER (eds): Immunologic Incompetence. Chicago, Year Book Medical, 1971, pp 3–13

45. Kohler PF, Farr RS: Elevation of cord over maternal IgG immunoglobulin—evidence for an active placental IgG transport. Nature 210:1070–1071, 1966

46. Thom H, McKay E, Gray DWG: Protein concentrations in the umbilical cord plasma of premature and mature infants. Clin Sci 33:433–444, 1967

47. Bert T: Immunoglobulin levels in infants with low birth weights. Acta Paediatr Scand 57:369–376, 1968

48. Evans HE, Akpata SO, Glass L: Serum immunoglobulin levels in premature and full-term infants. Am J Clin Pathol 56:416–418, 1971

49. Yeung CY, Hobbs JR: Serum gamma G-globulin levels in normal, premature, post-mature and "small-for-dates" newborn babies. Lancet i:1167–1170, 1968

50. Papadatos C, Papaevangelou GH, Alexiou D, et al: Serum immunoglobulin G levels in small-for-dates newborn babies. Arch Dis Child 45:570–572, 1970

51. Amer J, Ott E, Ibbott FA, et al: The effect of monthly gamma-globulin administration on morbidity and mortality from infection in premature infants during the first year of life. Pediatrics 32:4–9, 1963

52. Hodes HL: Should the premature infant receive gamma globulin? Pediatrics 32:1–3, 1963

53. Stiehm ER: Fetal defense mechanism. Am J Dis Child 129:438–443, 1975

54. Martensson L, Fudenberg HH: Gm genes and IgG-globulin synthesis in the human fetus. J Immunol 94:514–520, 1965

55. Fudenberg HH, Fudenberg BR: Antibody to hereditary human gamma-globulin (Gm) factor resulting from maternal–fetal incompatibility. Science 145:170–171, 1964

56. Steinberg AG: Progress in the study of genetically determined gamma globulin types (the Gm and Inv groups). Prog Med Genet 2:1–33, 1962

57. Alford CA, Schaefer J, Blankenship WJ, et al: A correlative immunologic, microbiologic and clinical approach to the diagnosis of acute and chronic infections in newborn infants. N Engl J Med 277:437–449, 1967

58. Miller MJ, Sunshine PJ, Remington JS: Quantitation of cord serum

IgM and IgA as a screening procedure to detect congenital infection—results in 5 or 6 infants. J Pediatr 75:1287–1291, 1969

59. Dent PB, Finkel A, Iturzaeta N, et al: Intrauterine infection and cord immunoglobulin M-1. Analysis of methods of assay and levels of immunoglobulin M in normal newborns. Can Med Assoc J 106:889–893, 1972

60. Rowlands DT, Blakeslee D, Angola E: Acquired immunity in opossum (didelphis virginiana) embryos. J Immunol 112:2148–2153, 1974

61. Blaese RM, Henrichon M, Waldmann TA: Ontogeny of the immune response: The afferent limb, abstracted. Fed Proc 29:699, 1970

62. Braun W, Lasky LF: Antibody formation to newborn mice initiated through adult macrophages, abstracted. Fed Proc 26:642, 1967

63. Argyris BF: Role of macrophages in immunological maturation. J Exp Med 128:459–467, 1968

64. Blaese RM, Lawrence EC: Development of macrophage function and the expression of immunocompetence, in Cooper MD, Dayton DH (eds): Development of Host Defenses. New York, Raven Press, 1977, p 201

4

The Immune Response of the Neonate

As reviewed in the previous two chapters, the T- and B-cell systems have developed a degree of functional integrity by the time of birth. While much information exists on the individual T- and, particularly, B-cell responses during the neonatal period, almost no data are available on the functional interaction of T–B immunity.

MODULATING FACTORS

A unique aspect of the neonatal immune response derives from the presence within the newborn circulation of humoral and, perhaps, cellular factors derived from the mother during gesta-

43

tion. Chief among these factors are maternal antibodies, which have long been recognized to exert a suppressive effect upon neonatal antibody formation. In the case of antibodies that are effectively transferred across the placenta, for example, diphtheria, the immunosuppressive effects of maternal antibody may be substantial.[1-3] In the case of tetanus,[4] however, responses to antigen in infants 1 to 3 months of age were as appropriate as those in infants to whom antigen was administered between 6 and 14 months of age. This is presumably because tetanus antibodies are not transferred across the placenta as effectively as diphtheria antibodies.

Other humoral factors may exert an immunosuppressive effect upon neonatal antibody production. Nejedla suggested that bilirubin might be immunosuppressive.[5] Twelve infants with bilirubin levels greater than 15 mg/100 ml at birth who had not received exchange transfusions were followed for 1 year. Antibody responses to pertussis, diphtheria, tetanus, and *E. coli* were significantly less among these infants than among control groups of 25 normal infants and 40 infants with hyperbilirubinemia who had received exchange transfusions.

ACTIVE ANTIBODY PRODUCTION

The neonatal antibody response has been extensively studied. Interpretation of the data provided by these studies, however, leaves many unanswered questions.

In 1964, Smith and co-workers studied the responses of premature and term neonates to flagellar (H) and somatic (0) antigens of *Salmonella*.[6] They made the following specific observations:

1. Only those infants who had passively acquired low titers (1:20 or less) of anti-H antibody from their mothers showed a significant H agglutinin response upon administration of H antigen.
2. Most premature and term infants with maternally acquired titers of less than 1:20 showed a positive agglutinin response following administration of H antigen.
3. Older infants (over 13 days) showed a greater antibody response to H antigen than newborns.

4. Maturity did not seem to be a primary factor. Greater than 50 percent of the prematures developed H agglutinin titers of at least 1:10 by day 7 following immunization, and by day 14, this number had risen to 80 percent. Titers of H agglutinin were, in many cases, comparable to those measured in adults. In support of these findings, Rothberg found that the antibody response of premature infants to oral bovine serum albumin was equivalent to that of term infants,[5] suggesting that the interval from birth is more important than size or somatic maturation.

5. H agglutinin response was heterogeneous with respect to antibody class. The sequence observed was comparable to that seen in the adult. The first antibodies were macroglobulins, presumably IgM. Subsequent antibodies were found in the IgG fraction. The only substantive difference between the heterogeneity of the neonatal and adult responses was in the kinetics of the IgM → IgG phase. While adults showed IgG activity within 5 to 15 days, only IgM was found in the neonates for as long as 20 to 30 days following immunization. The period of prolonged IgM shift lasted until 6 months of age, which is comaprable to data of other investigators.[7-15]

6. Response to *Salmonella* 0 antigen in prematures and neonates differed significantly from that observed in adults. A positive response to 0 antigen was rarely elicited in infants, while 0 agglutinins appeared within 14 days in a titer range of 1:5 to 1:160 in all immunized adults. Positive 0 agglutinin responses were not observed in infants under the age of 3 to 9 months.

One need look no further than to the above studies to appreciate the spectrum of unknowns of the host repsonse in the neonate. A number of possible explanations may be offered to explain the differences between H and O antigen response in neonates. Smith and co-workers[6] suggested that either the O antigen was less effective than the H antigen in eliciting a response in newborns or that the assay technique for measurement of O agglutinins was less sensitive than that for H agglutinins.[16] Alternative explanations may be proposed, including (1) a defect of macrophage or phagocyte processing of O antigen and (2) an excess or imbalance of suppressor T cells during the neonatal period. T-cell modulation of B-cell differentiation appears to be by suppression in neonatal mice[17] and in man.[18] The effects of helper

T cells may be masked by excessive suppressor-cell activity. The relative ease of establishing tolerance in the newborn[17] and the deficient antibody response to pneumococcal or meningococcal polysaccharide antigens during infancy[19] may be due to dominance of suppressor T cells.[20,21]

Neonatal antibody responses to other antigens have been less extensively studied. Available data, however, differ somewhat from the Smith studies. With diphtheria toxoid, Dancis and co-workers found only a small percentage of full-term and premature infants immunized during the first week of life who developed diphtheria antitoxin within 1 month.[22]

Provenzano and co-workers found that 21 of 22 neonates immunized with pertussis vaccine during the first 14 hours of life had inadequate responses.[23] Upon reimmunization, 75 percent of these infants had a poor response up to the age of 15 months. Other studies have found a diminished antibody response by neonates to diphtheria toxoid,[24] inactivated poliomyelitis vaccine,[25] or pertussis whole bacterial vaccine.[26]

PASSIVE IMMUNITY

IgG

Passively acquired maternal IgG antibodies confer protection upon the newborn against a wide variety of organisms, including measles, rubella, meningococci, streptococci, and *Hemophilus influenzae.*[27] Only partial protection is provided toward organisms against which high titers of protective IgG do not persist, such as vaccinia, varicella, pertussis, tetanus, and diphtheria. Only mothers who have recently been infected or immunized with organisms of the latter group are likely to provide protection to their infants. Antibodies against gram-negative organisms such as *E. coli* and *Salmonella* reside primarily within the IgM class and do not cross the placenta. There are, however, some IgG antibodies against somatic antigens of gram-negative organisms, thereby affording a degree of protection to most infants.[28] A relative deficiency of IgM was thought to play a major role in explaining enhanced susceptibility to infection of neonates, particularly toward gram-negative organisms.[29] Reexamination of this point, however, suggests that IgM deficiency may be only one factor in the equation (see section on Opsonins).

IgG SUBCLASSES

Four subclasses of IgG have been recognized: IgG_1, IgG_2, IgG_3, and IgG_4. Each subclass has distinct antigenic, metabolic, and presumably functional properties, although the latter have not been well defined. Placental transfer of all four IgG subclasses appears to be complete by term, although some question remains on transfer of IgG_2. In studies of pooled neonatal and adult sera, Wang and co-workers found a decrease in placental transport of IgG_2.[30] If so, this would result in a clinically significant decrease of IgG_2, which contains many antibodies against polysaccharide antigens. In the same studies, an IgG heavy chain present in pooled neonatal sera was not present in adult IgG_1, leading the authors to hypothesize a new subclass of IgG. This was termed IgF and was presumably specific for the fetus and endogenously synthesized. In studies on 115 maternal and 128 fetal sera, mostly maternal–fetal pairs (not pooled), however, Morrell and co-workers found no deficiency of IgG_2 in cord blood.[31] The presence of IgG_2 in cord blood was confirmed by assays for GM (23), a genetic marker for IgG_2. In all instances in which the maternal sera had GM (23) activity, the corresponding cord sera also contained GM (23) of equal activity.

Considerable heterogeneity of IgG subclass levels is observed in the first 2 years of life.[32] During the neonatal period, levels of all IgG subclasses decrease sharply, but IgG_3 falls off most rapidly, decreasing to approximately 50 percent of term levels by 30 days postnatally.

IgM

Synthesis of IgM occurs rapidly after birth. The levels rise rapidly during days 4 to 7 of life,[33] perhaps as a result of antigenic stimulation by intestinal colonization.

IgA

IgA first appears in neonatal sera at an average age of 15 days (range 5 to 23 days).[34] IgA has been detected in several sites prior to appearance in serum. McKay and Thom found IgA in tears of newborn infants between 10 to 20 days of age.[35] In saliva, Haworth and Dilling found IgA initially at 2 to 3 weeks of age, preceding its appearance in serum.[36]

Evidence has been summarized supporting the secretory nature of this IgA.[27] Secretory IgA has a larger molecular weight (400,000) than does serum IgA and an additional antigenic piece, the secretory component, synthesized by glandular epithelial cells.[37] Secretory IgA is synthesized in plasma cells found adjacent to epithelial surfaces[38] and functions as a dimmer of IgA linked together by a polypeptide chain called a "J" (joining) chain. Remington and Schaefer found free secretory component in the urine of newborn premature infants in the absence of urinary IgA.[39]

IgD

IgD is usually absent in cord blood. Evans and co-workers detected IgD in 8 percent of newborns (84 studied).[40] Berg found IgD in only 1 of 64 premature infants.[41]

IgE

Little, if any, IgE crosses the placenta.[42–44] Reaginic activity, as measured by skin testing with anti-IgE serum, was not detected in 29 of 34 newborns,[44] but the skin tests became positive at a mean age of 21.7 days. (As discussed later in this chapter, however, the significance of skin tests in neonates is unclear.)

Stevenson and co-workers, utilizing radioimmunoassay, found a mean cord IgE level of 39.1 ng/ml compared with mean maternal levels of 177.2 ng/ml.[44] Johannson found a mean cord IgE level of 36.3 ng/ml compared with a maternal level of 286 ng/ml.[45] Bazaral and co-workers, using a modified radioimmunoassay, found mean cord serum levels of IgE to be 2.1 units/

ml (0.45 units IgE equivalent to approximately 1 ng), with mean maternal levels of 92.4 units/ml.[46] More recently, Orgel and co-workers found neonatal levels of IgE ranging from 0 to 10 units/ml.[47] In their study, the relationship of serum IgE levels to the development of atopic disease was also analyzed. Elevation of serum IgE levels at or before 1 year of age was highly correlated with atopic disease in the first 2 years of life. The elevation preceded the manifestation of atopy.

CELLULAR IMMUNE RESPONSE

The Neonatal Skin Test Response

An extensive literature describes attempts to characterize T-cell function in neonates through assays of various types of skin test reactivity. As we shall now review, however, the skin test depends upon a complex set of interactions including, but not solely dependent upon, T-cell function. Hence, a negative skin test does not necessarily imply deficient T-cell function.

INTRADERMAL AND PATCH TESTING

In 1929, Freund found negative skin tests in newborn guinea pigs injected with tubercle baccili.[48] Strauss[49] and Tschertkow[50] found that newborn infants were less readily sensitized than adults to, respectively, *Rhus* extract and *Salmonella* extract. Gaisford found that Mantoux tests become positive within 14 to 21 days following BCG immunization in infants but that the intensity of the reaction was less than that in the adult.[51] With contact sensitivity, Epstein found that infants under 1 year of age were less readily sensitized than adults to pentadecyl catechol, a *Rhus* extract.[52]

Uhr and co-workers studied the skin response in premature and term infants to 2, 4-dinitrochlorobenzene (DNCB).[53] Ten premature infants (average birth weight, 1255 gm) and 5 term infants were immunized percutaneously with 0.02–0.04 ml of 10% DNCB in acetone during the first week of life. Patch testing of all children with 0.01 M DNCB was carried out at 2 to 4 weeks following sensitization. All the control subjects, 2 of the 5 term infants, and 3 of the 10 prematures showed positive skin responses. The lesions showed basically the same histologic results as found in contact-type hypersensitivity in the adult. Response to sensitization bore no relationship to weight of the premature or term infants. The authors concluded that delayed hypersensitivity can be induced during the neonatal period but, partly as a result of a diminished inflammatory response, may yield inconsistent results.

HOMOGRAFT REJECTION

Fowler studied 12 neonates who had received exchange transfusions for hyperbilirubinemia.[59] Each infant received a skin allograft with skin from their respective blood donor. The freshness of the donor blood administered affected the allograft survival. Skin grafts survived for prolonged periods when fresh blood had been used in the exchange transfusion, while grafts placed on infants who had received blood stored for more than 48 hours prior to exchange were rapidly rejected. It is conceivable that a higher concentration of lymphocytes was present in the fresh blood and that a degree of tolerance to the skin grafts had been induced. One 3-pound infant (equivalent to a gestational age of 32 weeks) rejected paternal skin by 12 days.

PASSIVE TRANSFER OF SENSITIZED CELLS

Substantial indication that skin reactivity of neonates may not be an accurate barometer of cell-mediated immunity is found in studies of passively transferred skin test reactivity. Sterzl and Hrubesova were able to passively transfer cutaneous reactivity to tuberculin with tuberculin-sensitized leukocytes of piglets to tuberculin-negative adult pigs, even though the piglet donors were themselves skin-test negative.[55] In other studies in humans, Warwick and co-workers[56] and Fowler and co-workers[57] were unable to passively transfer cutaneous reactivity against several antigens to newborns by administering leukocytes from older children and adults with positive skin reactivity for the same antigens. Although Schlange was able to transfer tuberculin reactivity from tuberculin-positive adults to newborns, his studies employed exchange transfusions.[58] It is possible that other substances or cells besides T cells present in whole blood could account for this transfer.

CUTANEOUS INFLAMMATION

Fireman tested 1- to 2-day-old neonates, born of mothers with positive or negative PPD responses.[59] The infants were tested for reactivity to PPD by in vivo (intracutaneous) and in vitro (leuko-cyte stimulation) methods. None of the infants initially showed reactivity to PPD by either method. Infants then received either leukocytes or leukocyte transfer factor from PPD-positive mothers. Lymphocytes subsequently obtained from the infants showed increased in vitro response to PPD by blast transforma-tion or incorporation of ^{3}H-thymidine into nucleoprotein. By con-trast, the same infants showed no in vivo reactivity to PPD. Leukocytes from 3 infants who had failed to show a positive skin test upon passive sensitization were, however, found to passively transfer cutaneous tuberculin reactivity to 2 of 3 PPD-negative adult recipients. Finally, BCG was administered to the passively sensitized infants and to a group of normal nonsensitized infants. In vivo cutaneous and in vitro leukocyte responses to PPD were the same in both groups. In vitro leukocyte responses to PPD preceded the development of positive skin tests by 1 to 3 weeks. These data thus demonstrated that antigen-responsive lympho-cytes may be present in the newborn despite a negative skin test reaction.

Schwartz and Osburn studied the inflammatory response to turpentine, bacterial lipopolysaccharides, heat-killed *Staph-ylococcus aureus,* and immune complexes in fetal monkeys.[60] The earliest observed reaction was in a 90-day-old fetus, 24 hours following the injection of turpentine. Fetal reactivity to irritants differed from that in the adult: (1) the earliest cell response in fetuses was a mononuclear cell infiltrate; (2) PMN were absent or decreased in young fetuses, and when present in older fetuses, responded sluggishly; (3) edema and fibrin were absent in lesions of early fetal life.

Dixon[61] found deficient edema formation in fetal rats sub-jected to thermal trauma, as did Schwartz[62] following adminis-tration of histamine and bradykinin to fetal and newborn mon-keys.

Hess[63] found no deficiency in fibrin clot formation by day 1 in fetuses following a wound, but Weiss and Matoltsy[64] found defi-cient epithelialization in chicken embryo wounds which they at-tributed to defective plasma scab formation.

Inflammation following dermal infection with pneumococci

was studied by Seto and Drachman.[65] Weanling rats showed (1) increased incidence of bacteremia and death; (2) delayed migration of leukocytes and mononuclear cells; and (3) poor localization and increased spreading of bacteria.

Response of neonatal skin to irritants and ability to localize inflammation is also deficient in comparison to adults.[66]

INFLAMMATORY CYCLE

In 1955, Rebuck and Crowley described a procedure for studying in vivo inflammation that is commonly known as the "skin window."[67] In this procedure, a superficial abrasion is created on the skin and a cover slip placed over the inflammatory site. By periodically changing the cover slip, a normal sequence of cellular emigration can be identified. In normal adults, polymorphonuclear leukocytes predominate in the first 4 to 12 hours, followed by a gradual shift to a mononuclear response.

The neonatal inflammatory cycle is not particularly remarkable, although two abnormalities have been identified: (1) the shift from a predominately granulocytic to monocytic phase is slower and less intense in neonates than in adults,[66,68,69] and (2) an abnormality of the eosinophil response in neonates may exist. Eitzman and Smith found a high percentage of eosinophils in the 2- and 4-hour exudate of neonates over 24 hours of age but not in those under 24 hours of age.[66] Bullock and co-workers, however, found increased percentages of eosinophils in only 13 of 61 infants.[69] They suggested that these 13 infants might represent a subgroup with a possible allergic diathesis.

T-CELL FUNCTION

As reviewed above, the vast majority of work on presumed T-cell function in neonates has involved cutaneous parameters that probably reflect developmental immaturity of inflammatory components (Chapters 5 and 6) more than T-cell deficiency. There remains a wide gap in our understanding of the T-cell response in neonates. Almost no information is available on specific T-cell subsets or T-cell products such as lymphokines (Chapter 2). These will, no doubt, be active areas of research in the near future.

Some data are available on T-cell functions in the human neonate. Most reports have described responsiveness of cord blood lymphocytes to PHA stimulation. Data from such studies are contradictory, owing in part to methodologic differences but probably also to incomplete understanding and correction for individual lymphocyte subpopulations. Standardization of total numbers of lymphocytes in such assays may not ensure consistent numbers of individual types of T cells or other peripheral blood cells affecting such responses. Cord blood lymphocytes undergo a considerably greater degree of spontaneous or unstimulated transformation than do adult lymphocytes. This has been measured by either blast transformation or incorporation of radiolabeled thymidine.[70-72] Alford and co-workers observed enhanced spontaneous thymidine incorporation in lymphocytes up to 3 months of age[73] (Chapter 2).

Buckley and co-workers evaluated T-cell mediated IgE immune responses to pollen allergen in various groups of subjects, including 4 normal newborns.[74] An important role for T cells in regulating IgE antibody responses to antigens has been demonstrated.[75] Cultured lymphocytes were exposed to purified ragweed antigens E, K, and Ra-3, and DNA synthetic responses were measured by ^{3}H-thymidine incorporation. Newborn lymphocytes showed a vigorous response to these purified pollen allergens, as did lymphocytes from nonatopic normal, atopic, and hypogammaglobulinemic subjects. The authors suggested either that ragweed pollen antigens are ubiquitous and lead to cell-mediated responsiveness in all subjects with intact cell-mediated immunity or that they may have mitogenic properties in addition to their known antigenicity. If the first postulate proves correct, then this would be evidence for an intact T-cell response in normal newborns.

REFERENCES

1. Smith T: Active immunity produced by so-called balanced or neutral mixtures of diphtheria toxin and anti-toxin. J Exp Med 11:241–256, 1909
2. Mason JH, Robinson M, Christensen PA: The active immunization

of guinea pigs passively immunized with homologous antitoxin serum. J Hyg (Camb) 53:172–179, 1955

3. Greengard J, Bernstein H:.Passive immunity in infants and their response to diphtheria toxoid. JAMA 105:341–342, 1935

4. Cooke JV: Antibody formation in early infancy against diphtheria and tetanus toxoids. J Pediatr 33:141–146, 1948

5. Nejedla A: The development of immunological factors in infants with hyperbilirubinemia. Pediatrics 45:102–104, 1970

6. Smith RT, Eitzman DV, Catlin ME, et al: Development of the immune response. Response of newborn and mature humans to salmonella vaccines. Pediatrics 33:163–183, 194

7. Rothberg RM: Immunoglobulins and specific antibody synthesis during the first weeks of life of premature infants. J Pediatr 75:151–156, 1953

8. Bridges RA, Condie RM, Zak SJ et al: The morphologic basis of antibody formation development during the neonatal period. J Lab Clin Med 53:331–357, 1959

9. Zak SJ, Good RA: Immunochemical studies of human serum gamma globulines. J Clin Invest 38:579–586, 1959

10. Bauer DC, Stavitsky AB: On the different molecular forms of antibody synthesized by rabbits during the early response to a single infection of protein and cellular antigens. Proc Natl Acad Sci USA 47:1667–1680, 1961

11. Uhr JW, Dancis J, Franklin EC, et al: The antibody response to bacteriophage ϕX 174 in newborn premature infants. J Clin Invest 41:1509–1513, 1962

12. Fink CW, Miller WE Jr, Dorward B et al: The formation of macroglobulin antibodies. II. Studies on neonatal infants and older children. J Clin Invest 41:1422–1428, 1962

13. LoSpalutto J, Miller WE Jr, Dorward B: Formation of macroglobulin antibodies. I. Studies on adult humans. J Clin Invest 41:1415–1421, 1962

14. Benedict AA, Brown R, Ayengar R: Physical properties of antibody to bovine serum albumin as demonstrated by hemagglutination. J Exp Med 115:195–208, 1962

15. Bellanti JA, Etizman DV, Robbins JB et al: The development of the immune response: Studies of the agglutinin response to *Salmonella* flagellar antigens in the newborn rabbit. J Exp Med 117:479–496, 1963

16. Altemeier WA, Smith RT: Immunologic aspects of resistance in early life. Pediatr Clin North Am 12:663–686, 1965

17. Mosier DE, Johnson BM: Ontogeny of mouse lymphocyte function. II. Development of the ability to produce antibody is modulated by T lymphocytes. J Exp Med 141:216–226, 1975

18. Wu LYF, Blanco A, Cooper MD, et al: Ontogeny of B-lymphocytes differentiation induced by pokeweed mitogens. Clin Immunol Immunopathol 5:208–217, 1976

19. Goldschneider I, Lepow ML, Gotschlich EC: Immunogenicity of the group A and group C meningococcal polysaccharides in children. J Infect Dis 125:509–519, 1972

20. Hayward AR, Lawton AR: Induction of plasma cell differentiation of human fetal lymphocytes: evidence for functional immaturity of T and B cells. J Immunol 119:1213–1217, 1977

21. Olding LB, Benirschke K, Oldstone MBA: Inhibition of mitosis of lymphocytes from human adults by lymphocytes from human newborns. Clin Immunol Immunopath 3:79–89, 1974

22. Dancis J, Osborn JJ, Kunz HW: Studies of immunology of the newborn infant. IV. Antibody formation in the premature infant. Pediatrics 12:151–156, 1953

23. Provenzano RW, Wellerlow LH, Sullivan CL: Immunization and antibody response in the newborn infant—I. Pertussis inoculation within twenty-four hours of birth. N Engl J Med 273:959–965, 1965

24. Valhquist B: Response of infants to diphtheria immunization. Lancet i:16–18, 1949

25. Perkins FT, Yetts R, Gaisford W: Serological response of infants to poliomyelitis vaccine. Br Med J 2:68–71, 1958

26. Barrett CD Jr, McLean IW Jr, Jolner JG, et al: Multiple antigen immunization of infants against poliomyelitis, diphtheria, pertussis, and tetanus. Pediatrics 30:720–736, 1962

27. Miller ME, Stiehm ER: Phagocytic, opsonic, and immunoglobulin studies in newborns. Calif Med 119:43–63, 1973

28. Cohen IR, Norins LC: Antibodies of the IgG, IgM and IgA classes in newborn and adult sera reactive with gram-negative bacteria. J Clin Invest 47:1053–1062, 1968

29. Gitlin D, Rosen FS, Michael JG: Transient 19S gammaglobulin deficiency in the newborn infant, and its significance. Pediatrics 31:197–208, 1963

30. Wang AC, Faulk WP, Stuckey MA, et al: Chemical differences of adult, fetal and hypogammaglobulinemic IgG immunoglobulins. Immunochemistry 7:703–708, 1970

31. Morell A, Skvaril F, Van Loghem E, et al: Human IgG subclasses in maternal and fetal serum. Vox Sang 21:481–492, 1971

32. Morell A, Skvaril F, Hitzig WH, et al: IgG subclasses: Development of the serum concentrations in "normal" infants and children. J Pediatr 80:960–964, 1972

33. Allansmith M, McClellan BH, Butterworth M, et al: The development of immunoglobulin levels in man. J Pediatr 72:276–290, 1968

34. Stiehm ER, Fudenberg HH: Serum levels of immune globulins in health and disease—a survey. Pediatrics 37:715–727, 1966
35. McKay E, Thom H: Observations on neonatal tears. J Pediatr 75:1245–1256, 1969
36. Haworth JC, Dilling L: Concentration of gamma A-globulin serum, saliva and nasopharyngeal secretions of infants and children. J Lab Clin Med 67:922–933, 1966
37. Tomasi TB Jr: Secretory immunoglobulins. N Engl J Med 287:500–506, 1972
38. Bienenstock J: The local immune response. Am J Vet Res 36:488–491, 1975
39. Remington JS, Scheafer IA: Transport piece in the urines of premature infants. Nature 217:364–366, 1968
40. Evans HE, Akpata SO, Glass L: Serum immunoglobulin levels in premature and full-term infants. Am J Clin Pathol 56:416–418, 1971
41. Bert T: Immunoglobulin levels in infants with low birth weights. Acta Paediatr Scand 57:369–376, 1968
42. Klapper DG, Mendenhall HW: Immunoglobulin D concentration in pregnant women. J Immunol 107:912–915, 1971
43. Connell JT, Connell EB, Lidd D: Studies on the placental transfer of skin-sensitizing antibody, specific binding of a ragweed fraction, and immunoglobulins. J Allergy 39:57–63, 1967
44. Stevenson DD, Orgel HA, Hamburger RN, et al: Development of IgE in newborn human infants. J Allergy Clin Immunol 48:61–72, 1971
45. Johansson SGO: Serum IgND levels in healthy children and adults. Int Arch Allergy Immunol 34:1–8, 1968
46. Bazaral M, Orgel A, Hamburger RN: IgE levels in normal infants and mothers and an inheritance hypothesis. J Immunol 107:794–801, 1971
47. Orgel HA, Hamburger RN, Bazaral M: Development of IgE and allergy in infancy. J Allergy Clin Immunol 56:296–307, 1975
48. Freund J: The sensitiveness of tuberculous guinea pigs one month old to the toxicity of tuberculin. J Immunol 17:465–471, 1929
49. Strauss HW: Artificial sensitization of infants to poison ivy. J Allergy 2:137–144, 1931
50. Tschertkow L: Ueb er die Hautanergie bei Sauglingen. Z Immunitaetsforsch 64:407–412, 1929
51. Gaisford W: Protection of infants against tuberculosis. Br Med J 2:1164–1171, 1955
52. Epstein WL: Contact-type delayed hypersensitivity in infants and children: Induction of Rhus sensitivity. Pediatrics 27:51–53, 1961
53. Uhr JW, Dancis J, Neumann CG: Delayed-type hypersensitivity in

premature neonatal humans. Nature (London) 187:1130–1131, 1960

54. Fowler R Jr, Shubert WK, West CD: Acquired partial tolerance to homologous skin grafts in the human infant at birth. Ann NY Acad Sci 87:403–428, 1960

55. Sterzl J, Hrubesova M: Attempts to transfer tuberculin hypersensitivity to young rabbits. Folia Microbil (Praha) 4:60–61, 1959

56. Warwick WJ, Good RA, Smith RT: Failure of passive transfer of delayed hypersensitivity in the newborn human infant. J Lab Clin Med 56:139–147, 1960

57. Fowler R Jr, Shubert WK, West CD: Acquired partial tolerance to homologous skin grafts in the human infant at birth. Ann NY Acad Sci 87:403–428, 1960

58. Schlange H: Die passive ubertragung der tuberkulinhautempfindlichleit durch blutaustausch-transfusionen und die ubertragbarkeit erworbener tuberkulinnegativitat. Arch Kinderheilk 148:12–22, 1954

59. Fireman P, Kumate J, Gitlin D: Development of delayed hypersensitivity in neonates, abstracted. Section VIII. International Congress of Allergology, No. 211. Amsterdam, Excerpta Medica, 1970

60. Schwartz LW, Osburn BI: An ontogenetic study of the acute inflammatory reaction in the fetal rhesus monkey. I. Cellular response to bacterial and non-bacterial irritants. Lab Invest 31:441–453, 1974

61. Dixon JB: Inflammation in the foetal and neonatal rat: The local reaction to skin burns. J Pathol Bacteriol 80:73–82, 1960

62. Schwartz LW: Vascular leakage, a deficient response to exogenous histamine, 48/80, and bradykinin in the fetal and newborn monkey, abstracted. Fed Proc 33:604, 1974

63. Hess A: Reactions of mammalian fetal tissues to injury. II. Skin Anat Rec 119:435–447, 1954

64. Weiss P, Matoltsy AG: Would healing in chick embryos in vivo and in vitro. Dev Biol 1:302–326, 1959

65. Seto DWY, Drachman RH: Response to bacterial infection in the mature and immature animal abstracted. J Pediatr 69:978, 1966

66. Eitzman DV, Smith RT: The nonspecific inflammatory cycle in the neonatal infant. Am J Dis Child 97:326–334, 1959

67. Rebuck JW, Crowley JH: A method of studying leukocytic functions in vitro. Ann NY Acad Sci 59:757–805, 1955

68. Sheldon WH, Caldwell JBH: The mononuclear cell phase of inflammation in the newborn. Bull John Hopkins Hosp 112:258–269, 1963

69. Bullock JD, Robertson AF, Bodenbender MT, et al: Inflammatory response in the neonate re-examined. Pediatrics 44:58–61, 1969

70. Leiken S, Mochir-Fatemi F, Park K: Blast transformation of lymphocytes from newborn human infants. J Pediatr 72:510–517, 1968

71. Leiken S, Oppenheim JJ: Differences in transformation of adult and newborn lymphocytes stimulated by antigen, antibody and antigen-antibody complexes. Cell Immunol 1:468–475, 1970

72. Leiken S, Whang-Peng J, Oppenheim JJ: In vitro transformation of human cord blood lymphocytes by antigens, in Harris J (ed): Proceedings of the Fifth Leukocyte Culture Conference. New York, Academic Press, 1970

73. Alford RH, Cartwright BB, Sell SH: Ontogeny of human cell-mediated immunity: Age-related variation of in vitro infantile lymphocyte transformation. Infect Immunol 13:1170–1175, 1976

74. Buckley RH, Seymour F, Sanal SO, et al: Lymphocyte responses to purified ragweed alergens in vitro. 1. Proliferative responses in normal, newborn, agammaglobuline mil, and atopic subjects. J All Clin Immunol 59:70–78, 1977

75. Iada T, Okumura K: Regulation of homocytotropic antibody formation in the rat. v. Cell cooperation in the antihapten homocytotropic antibody response. J Immunol 107:1137–1145, 1971

5
Phagocytic Cells

DEVELOPMENTAL ASPECTS

Phagocytic cells constitute one of the most primitive host defense components. In protozoa, foreign substances are ingested and digested by the entire cell. In coelenterates such as hydra, two layers of cells are developed, with the entoderm serving as a fixed layer of phagocytes. In the sponge and other metazoa, a more abundant mesoderm is developed. The mobile cells of the mesoderm subserve a host defense function, while the fixed entodermal cells satisfy nutritional functions. A primitive circulatory system develops in lower animals. The presence therein of mobile phagocytic cells presumably provides a ready reserve to aid the slowly migrating tissue histiocytes.

Although a relatively late cell in phylogeny, the neutrophil is found early in human ontogeny.[1] In the early yolk sac stages of hematopoiesis, a few myelocytes and histiocytes are found in the blood islands. Granulocytopoiesis is evident during the second month of gestation, and lymphocytes appear in the third month. Monocytes first appear in the fourth month in the spleen and lymph nodes.

The appearance of alveolar macrophages has been studied in rabbits. Sieger[2] found on orderly increase in the number of functional alveolar macrophages during the last trimester of gestation, followed by a dramatic increase in number of cells immediately before birth and through 3 days postnatally.[2] Zeligs and co-workers obtained similar results except that the postnatal increase lasted through the first week.[3]

Structural properties in certain cells of the phagocytic system may differ in the newborn. Hardy and co-workers compared peritoneal macrophages from newborn mice with those of adults by light and electron microscopy.[4] A higher percentage of newborn mouse macrophages phagocytized turkey red blood cells as compared with macrophages derived from adult mice. Macrophages from newborn mice contained scarce rough endoplasmic reticulum in contrast to the well-developed reticular structure found in adult mouse macrophages. Surface negative charge analysis, using cationized ferritin for labeling anionic groups, revealed differences in density and location of the particles. The newborn mouse macrophages contained almost twice as many anionic groups per square micrometer compared with those of adults. In addition, the cationized ferritin particles were contiguous with the membrane of the newborn mouse macrophages, while on the adult cells the grains were located at a distance of about 100 Å from the outer dense line of the "unit membrane."

Ultrastructurally, the leukocytes and their granules of normal human newborns were similar to those of adults as studied by Morris and co-workers.[5]

FUNCTIONAL ASPECTS

The importance of phagocytic cells in body defenses was first emphasized by Elie Metchnikoff shortly before the turn of the century. Once he established that "the essential and primary element in typical inflammation consists in a reaction of the phagocytes against a harmful agent," it followed that deficiencies of the inflammatory response might lead to clinically significant impairments of host defenses. This hypothesis has been repeatedly confirmed over the past decade. Not only are disorders of phagocytic function widely recognized but, as we shall now see, functional immaturity of the phagocyte systems in neonates also contributes significantly to their impaired host defenses.

As discussed in Chapter 1, normal phagocyte function involves a number of distinct steps, including cell movement, cell recognition, ingestion, intracellular killing, and immunologic reactivity. We will review the development of each of these steps in neonatal polymorphonuclear leukocytes (PMN) and monocyte-macrophages (MNL).

Movement

The ability of phagocytes to move enables them to arrive at the site of injury or infection as a "line of defense" against invading microorganisms. Mechanisms of cell movement have been comprehensively studied in recent years.[6−9] In order to understand the significance of such studies in the neonate, the following points may be summarized:

1. Terminology of the field has recently been revised. Formerly, the term "chemotaxis" was applied to the general phenomenon of directed cell movement. In other words, a cell moving toward a gradient in an in vitro filter assay (see below) was said to be demonstrating chemotaxis, and all disorders of PMN movement detected through the use of such an assay were considered to be defects of chemotaxis. Active locomotion of cells depends upon intrinsic cellular mechanisms which are influenced by extrinsic factors. Such environmental stimuli may produce a change in the *direction* of locomotion (*chemotaxis*), or in the *speed* or frequency of locomotion of cells (*chemokinesis*).

2. An increasing number of substances have been shown to influence PMN movement, including serum factors, activated complement factors, coagulation-derived factors, bacterial metabolites, secretory products of sensitized lym-

phocytes and PMN, and denatured proteins. A number of
N-formylmethionyl peptides which can be synthesized in the
laboratory have also recently been shown to possess potent
effects upon PMN movement.

3.   While the mechanisms by which these factors initiate and
     mediate PMN movement are unclear, a number of responses
     have been identified following contact of phagocytes with
     such chemotactically active materials. These include (a) a
     rapid, brief depolarization, perhaps related to calcium
     and/or sodium influx, prolonged hyperpolarization, related
     to increased potassium permeability; (b) increased levels of
     cyclic guanosine monophosphate; (c) lysosomal enzyme re-
     lease; (d) increased glycolysis and hexose monophosphate
     shunt activity; (e) cell swelling; (f) increased numbers of
     microtubules; (g) presumed activation of contractile pro-
     teins. Blood leukocytes contain up to 10 percent of their total
     protein as actin and up to 3 percent of their protein as
     myosin (all reviewed in ref. 9).

4.   Methods for the in vitro measurement of cell movement re-
     main relatively imprecise, insensitive, and controversial.[9]
     Study of human PMN by the various methods suggests that
     no single method reflects all parameters of cell movement
     and that several types of measurements may therefore be
     necessary in order to adequately define PMN movement in a
     given patient. Among the more commonly used assays are
     (a) the "Boyden" assay in which the number of cells moving
     through a small-pore filter to a source of chemotactically
     active material are counted; (b) the direct visualization
     method of Wilkinson; (c) the visual assay system of Zigmond
     in which cells are observed under phase microscopy on a
     bridge across which a gradient of chemotactic factor is estab-
     lished; (d) migration of cells in agarose; (e) radiolabeled fil-
     ter techniques in which the Boyden assay is modified to
     count radiolabeled cells passing through the filter rather
     than using visual counting; (f) deformability of PMN by the
     technique of cell elastimetry; and (g) techniques measuring
     undirected locomotion, such as the capillary tube technique
     or the Boyden chamber in the absence of a chemotactic gra-
     dient.

5.   Separable mechanisms exist for the processes of directed
     migration and undirected, or random, migration. Although

the nature of these differences has not yet been established, disorders of PMN movement may be partially characterized by the study of PMN in both types of assay.[8]

PMN MOVEMENT

The chemotactic activity of neonatal leukocytes was compared with that of cells from adults in their ability to move toward chemotactic factors(s) generated from pooled, normal serum.[10] Neonatal leukocytes showed a consistent deficiency in their response to chemotactic factor(s) generated from incubation of fresh, pooled serum with *S. aureus, E. coli*, or antigen–antibody complexes. Pahwa and co-workers found that chemotaxis of cord blood PMN was decreased in comparison with PMN from healthy adults toward two different stimuli—endotoxin-activated normal serum and lymphocyte-derived chemotactic factor (LDCF).[11]

MNL MOVEMENT

Conflicting results have been obtained in studies of chemotaxis of neonatal monocytes. Klein and co-workers,[12] using an agarose migration technique, and Weston and colleagues[13] found neonatal monocytes to be less chemotactic than those from older infants or adults.

Kretschmer and co-workers found normal chemotaxis of monocytes from cord blood when stimulated by lymphokines generated by adult lymphocytes.[14] When stimulated by lymphokines derived from cord lymphocytes, however, newborn monocytes showed a decreased chemotactic response. The authors suggested that this poor response of cord monocytes might be due to an inhibitor of chemotaxis from neonatal lymphocytes for which only newborn monocytes have the appropriate receptor.

Pahwa and co-workers, however, utilizing a Boyden chamber technique, found monocyte chemotaxis in cord blood from healthy term infants to be normal to increased (115–126 percent) in comparison with that of healthy adult control subjects.[11] Cord serum was less inhibitory than pooled adult human serum for adult monocytes when the cells were suspended in 10 percent serum and tested for chemotaxis. No inhibition of chemotactic factors by either cord or adult sera was observed. As noted above, the same study demonstrated deficient chemotaxis of neonatal PMN. The authors suggested that the dissociation of chemotactic response of the two different phagocytic cells may represent a protective mechanism whereby one cell can compensate for a defect in the response of the other.

Recognition

Immune-dependent phagocytosis is presumably mediated by receptors on the phagocyte membrane. Attachment sites for the Fc portion of the immunoglobulin molecule and for C3 have been identified on human phagocytes. Little information is available on the development of receptors on neonatal phagocytes. Pross and co-workers found that the percentage of neutrophils bearing Fc and complement receptors was the same in both cord and adult blood.[15]

Phagocytosis

Phagocytosis is an energy-requiring process that involves the flow of hyaline pseudopods of cells around particles.[6,16] Recent evidence strongly suggests an active role for actin-myosin filaments in the mediation of cytoplasmic movement necessary for pseudopod formation.[7,17] The pseudopods surround and fuse about the attached particle in the formation of the phagosome. Cytoplasmic granules converge and fuse with the phagosome, and by the process of degranulation,[18] discharge their contents into the phagosome.

In the presence of concentrations of adult serum in excess of 10 percent, the phagocytic activity of isolated neonatal PMN is normal.[19-23] Phagocytic particles in these studies included *E. coli, S. aureus* 502A, *Serratia marcescens, S. pyogenes, Diplococcus pneumoniae,* and *Pseudomonas aeruginosa.*

By contrast, several studies have demonstrated that phagocytic activity in neonatal PMN is less than that of adult PMN when performed in the presence of serum concentrations of less than 10 percent. Matoth, in 1952, showed that phagocytosis of starch granules by washed leukocytes from cord blood of term infants was equal to that of adult blood when the tests were performed in the presence of a 1:3 dilution of adult serum.[24] When the adult serum was diluted to 1:6 or 1:12, however, cord PMN showed decreased phagocytic activity compared with that of adult

PMN. This difference was greatest at serum concentrations of 2.5 to 3 percent. Miller found identical results with a system utilizing baker's yeast as the phagocytic particle.[25]

Under stress conditions, therefore, the neonatal PMN may be deficient in phagocytic activity. In support, Forman and Stiehm found 6 of 9 term infants with a variety of underlying clinical disorders to have deficient phagocytic activity of their PMN.[19]

In premature infants, phagocytic activity of PMN was reported as normal by several investigators[19,26] and as mildly deficient by others.[27,28] All these studies were performed with serum concentrations in excess of 10 percent, however.

Bactericidal Activity

Bactericidal activity in normal PMN results from a series of biochemical events. Following phagocytosis, PMN show increased oxygen consumption, oxidation of glucose via the hexose monophosphate shunt, and the generation of hydrogen peroxide.

This burst of metabolic activity is triggered by phagocytosis, which appears to activate an enzyme (presumably an oxidase) either on, or closely associated with, the cell surface. This results in the transfer of one electron to oxygen, which forms an unstable free radical termed superoxide anion (O_2^-). Two superoxide radicals can interact spontaneously and form hydrogen peroxide (H_2O_2), and continued interaction between H_2O_2 and O_2 forms hydroxyl radical (.OH), a potent oxidizing agent. Transfer of energy from O_2 perhaps to an unstable, excited species termed singlet oxygen results in a burst of luminescence and is probably the major contributor to NBT reduction.

Additional microbicidal activities result from the discharge of contents of cytoplasmic granules into the phagosome. The precise role played by such materials as phagocytin, lysozyme, and lactoferrin in PMN bactericidal activity or activities remains to be determined.[18]

PMN BACTERICIDAL ACTIVITY

As in phagocytosis, variable results have been obtained in studies of bactericidal activity of neonatal PMN. Cocchi and Marianelli studied bactericidal activity toward viable *P. aeruginosa* and found that the bactericidal rate of premature leukocytes was equal to those of controls at 90 minutes but lagged at 3 hours.[26] This defect was serum independent. Coen and co-workers[20] found decreased bactericidal activity in leukocytes from 9 of 25 term infants within the first 12 hours of life.

By contrast, other investigators have found normal bactericidal activities in neonatal PMN. Forman and Stiehm found normal killing of bacteria by PMN from normal term and low birth weight infants.[19] Park and co-workers found normal staphylocidal activity in neonatal PMN.[21] McCracken and Eichenwald found normal bactericidal activities of PMN from 18 term and premature infants against *S. aureus* 502A, *E. coli*, and *P. aeruginosa.*[23]

The ability of neonatal PMN to kill *Candida* may be decreased, even in the presence of pooled adult sera.[29]

As with phagocytosis, bactericidal activity of neonatal PMN may not be normal in "stress" situations. Thus, Wright and co-workers found decreased leukocyte bactericidal activities in infants with sepsis, meconium aspiration, respiratory distress syndrome, hyperbilirubinemia, and premature rupture of the membrane.[30]

MNL BACTERICIDAL ACTIVITY

Monocyte bactericidal activities in neonates were found to be normal by Kretschmer and co-workers[14] and by Orlowski and colleagues.[31] In the latter study, the monocytes of both infants and adults were significantly less active than were their PMN, but the bactericidal capacity did not differ appreciably between newborn and adult cells of either type. Deficient MNL killing in neonates has been reported by Bellanti and co-workers.[32]

Immunologic Reactivity

Macrophages play a role in the modulation of antibody response to a variety of antigens. Although the precise mechanisms by which macrophages interact with the T- and B-cell systems are unclear, it is likely that such interactions derive at least in part from "antigen processing" by the macrophage. The degree, if any, to which the human PMN participates in this process in unknown.

Some of the data in this area have been reviewed (Chapter 3), and it was noted that adult macrophages may reconstitute deficient antibody production in neonatal rats. Further evidence that neonatal macrophages are deficient in immunologic reactivity is provided by the findings that they could not reconstitute an antibody response to *Shigella* in adult x-irradiated recipients,[33] while transfer of adult peritoneal macrophages to such recipients resulted in an enhanced antibody response.[34] In another study, mouse macrophages, within the first 5 days after birth, exhibited a qualitatively deficient cellular immune response as compared with that of adult mice.[35] The impaired immunologic function cannot be simply attributed to phagocytosis, since macrophages capable of phagocytosis have been shown to exist already in the embryo.[36]

Milgrom and Shore reported normal neonatal monocyte function in immune serum, antibody-dependent cellular toxicity (Chapter 2). The effector cells in this process vary with different target cells and experimental designs. When antibody-coated human red blood cells serve as target cells mediating antibody-dependent cellular cytotoxicity, monocytes act as the mononuclear effector cell. In such a system, monocytes of newborn infants demonstrated full activity as compared with adult monocytes as effectors in antibody-dependent cellular cytotoxicity.

Deformability

Utilizing the technique of cell elastimetry, Miller has shown that neonatal PMN have markedly decreased deformability over control PMN—i.e., are much more rigid cells.[37] In this technique, cells to be studied are maneuvered to the orifice of micropipettes, and the amount of negative pressure required to aspirate the cell into the pipette is determined under direct microscopic visualization. The increased rigidity of the neonatal PMN as determined in these studies may contribute significantly to the impaired chemotaxis and the more subtle deficiency of phagocytosis in their cells.

Metabolic Activities

Since metabolic processes underlie normal phagocytic functions, it comes as no surprise that the metabolic status of neonatal phagocytes has been widely investigated. Despite this, there is relatively little consistent data.

PMN METABOLIC ACTIVITIES

Donnell and co-workers[38] and Coen and colleagues[20] found decreased activity of hexose monophosphate shunt pathway in phagocytizing PMN of neonates compared with adult PMN. Park and co-workers found that resting-state neonatal neutrophils consumed twice as much oxygen as did maternal neutrophils.[21] Following phagocytosis, however, these authors observed the same increase in oxygen consumption and glucose utilization in neonatal and maternal PMN. Studies under both resting conditions and during infection suggested that neonatal neutrophils had less of an increase in the hexosemonophosphate shunt pathway but utilized glucose and oxygen in similar amounts to those seen in adult PMN following phagocytosis.[20,21,38,39]

Reduction of nitroblue tetrazolium (NBT) has been studied in neonatal PMN with variable results.[23,40,41] Park and co-workers found increased NBT reduction by cord blood PMN,[21] while Bellanti and co-workers found decreased reduction.[42] McCracken and Eichenwald found normal NBT reduction in PMN from 41 infants ranging in age from 2 hours to 71 days.[23] In explanation of these discrepancies, Bellanti and co-workers have suggested that leukocyte glucose-6-phosphate dehydrogenase (G6PD) activity decays at a significantly greater rate in newborn than in adult PMN.[43] NBT reduction by cord blood monocytes was found equal to that of adult monocytes by Kretschmer and co-workers.[44]

MNL METABOLIC ACTIVITIES

Das and co-workers compared glycolytic metabolism of cord blood mononuclear cells from 60 term and 8 premature infants with that of mononuclear cells from normal adults and pregnant women immediately before delivery.[45] The neonatal mononuclear cells were deficient in two glycolytic energy-producing enzymes, phosphoglycerate kinase and pyruvate kinase. Cells from the premature infants were more severely decreased in these enzymes and were also deficient in adenylate kinase. The mononuclear cell preparations contained 10 to 20 percent monocytes. As noted by the authors, ". . . the metabolic changes observed may reflect an immaturity of the monocyte population, rather than an alteration in the lymphocytes." Future studies should clarify this point.

REFERENCES

1. Bierman HR: Cited in MacFarlane RG, Robb-Smith AHT (eds): Functions of the Blood. New York, Academic Press, 1961, pp 350–418
2. Sieger L: Pulmonary alveolar macrophages in pre- and post-natal rabbits. J Reticuloendothel Soc (in press)
3. Zeligs BJ, Nerukar LS, Bellanti JA et al: Maturation of the rabbit alveolar macrophage during animal development. I. Perinatal influx into alveoli and ultrastructural differentiation. Pediatr Res 11:197–208, 1977
4. Hardy B, Skutelsky E, Globerson A, et al: Ultrastructural differences between macrophages of newborn and adult mice. J Reticuloendothel Soc 19:291–299, 1976
5. Morris RB, Nichols BA, Bainton DF: Ultrastructural and peroxidase cytochemistry of normal human leukocytes at birth. Dev Biol 44:223–238, 1975
6. Stossel TP: Phagocytosis: Recognition and ingestion. Semin Hematol 12:83–116, 1975
7. Stossel TP, Hartwig JH: Interaction of actin, myosin, and a new actin-binding protein of rabbit pulmonary macrophage II. Role in cytoplasmic movement and phagocytosis. J Cell Biol 68:602–619, 1976
8. Miller ME: Pathology of chemotaxis and random mobility. Semin Hematol 12:59–82, 1975
9. Quie PG, Gallin JI (eds): Leukocyte Chemotaxis. New York, Raven Press, 1978
10. Miller ME: Chemotactic function in the human neonate: Humoral and cellular aspects. Pediatr Res 5:487–492, 1971
11. Pahwa S, Pahwa R, Grimes E, et al: Cellular and humoral components of monocyte and neutrophil chemotaxis in cord blood. Pediatr Res 11:677–680, 1977
12. Klein RB, Fischer TJ, Gard SE, et al: Decreased mononuclear and polymorphonuclear chemotaxis in newborns. Pediatrics 60(4):467–472, 1977
13. Weston WL, Carson BS, Barkin RM, et al: Monocyte-macrophage function in the newborn. Clin Res 28:182A, 1976
14. Kretschmer RR, Stewardson BB, Papiernialo CK, et al: Chemotactic and bactericidal capacities of human newborn monocytes. J Immunol 117:1303–1307, 1976
15. Pross SH, Hallock JA, Armstrong R, et al: Complement and Fc receptors on cord blood and adult neutrophils. Pediatr Res 11:135–157, 1977
16. Wilkinson PC: Recognition and response in mononuclear and granular phagocytes. Clin Exp Immunol 25:355–366, 1976

17. Boxer LA, Stossel TP: Interactions of actin, myosin and an actin-binding protein of chronic myelogenous leukemia leukocytes. J Clin Invest 57:964–976, 1976

18. Ryan GB, Majno G: Acute inflammation. Am J Pathol 86:185–276, 1977

19. Forman ML, Stiehm ER: Impaired opsonic activity but normal phagocytosis in low-birth-weight infants. N Engl J Med 281:926–931, 1969

20. Coen R, Grush O, Kauder E: Studies of bactericidal activity and metabolism of the leukocyte in full-term neonates. J Pediatr 75:400–406, 1969

21. Park BH, Holmes B, Good RA: Metabolic activities in leukocytes of newborn infants. J Pediatr 76:237–241, 1970

22. Dossett JH, Williams RC Jr, Quie PG: Studies on interaction of bacteria, serum factors and polymorphonuclear leukocytes in mothers and newborns. Pediatrics 44:49–57, 1969

23. McCracken GH, Eichenwald HF: Leukocyte function and the development of opsonic and complement activity in the neonate. Am J Dis Child 121:120–126, 1971

24. Matoth Y: Phagocytic and ameboid activities of the leukocytes in the newborn infant. Pediatrics 9:748–754, 1952

25. Miller ME: Phagocytosis in the newborn infant: Humoral and cellular factors. J Pediatr 74:255–259, 1969

26. Cocchi P, Marianelli L: Phagocytosis and intracellular killing of *Pseudomonas aeruginosa* in premature infants. Helv Paediatr Acta 22:110–118, 1967

27. Miyamoto K: Phagocytic activity of leucocytes in premature infants. I. Comparison of the phagocytic activity of leucocytes between premature infants and full term infants. Hiroshima J Med Sci 14:9–17, 1965

28. Gluck L, Silverman WA: Phagocytosis in premature infants. Pediatrics 20:951–957, 1957

29. Xanthou M: Leukocyte blood picture in healthy full-term and premature babies during neonatal period. Arch Dis Child 45:242–249, 1970

30. Wright WC Jr, Ank BJ, Herbert J, et al: Decreased bactericidal activity of leukocytes of stressed newborn infants. Pediatrics 56:579–584, 1975

31. Orlowski JP, Sieger L, Anthony BF: Bactericidal capacity of monocytes of newborn infants. J Pediatr 89:797–801, 1976

32. Bellanti JA, Nerurkar L, Zeligs B, et al: Postnatal development of rabbit alveolar macrophages, abstracted. J Reticuloendothel Soc 18(6):27b, 1975

33. Hardy B. Globerson A, Danon D: Ontogenic development of the reactivity of macrophages to antigenic stimulation. Cell Immunol 9:282–288, 1973

34. Gallily R, Feldman M: The role of macrophages in the induction of antibody in x-irradiated animals. Immunology 12:197–206, 1967

35. Yang HY, Skinsnes OK: Peritoneal macrophage response in neonatal mice. J Reticuloendothel Soc 14:181–191, 1973

36. Cline MJ, Moore MAS: Embryonic origin of the mouse macrophage. Blood 39:842–849, 1972

37. Miller ME: Developmental maturation of human neutrophil motility and its relationship to membrane deformability, in Bellanti JA, Dayton DS (eds): The Phagocytic Cell in Host Resistance. New York, Raven Press, 1975, pp 295–307

38. Donnell GN, Ng WG, Hodgman JE, et al: Galactose metabolism in the newborn infant. Pediatrics 39:829–837, 1967

39. Anderson DC, Pickering LK, Fergin RD: Leukocyte function in normal and infected neonates. J Pediatr 85:420–425, 1974

40. Humbert JR, Kurtz ML, Hathaway WE: Increased reduction of nitroblue tetrazolium by neutrophils of newborn infants. Pediatrics 45:125–128, 1969

41. Cocchi P, Mori S, Becattini A: NBT tests in premature infants. Lancet ii:1425–1427, 1969

42. Bellanti JA, Cantz BE, Yang MC, et al: Leukocyte maturation: G-6-PD activity and NBT dye reduction, abstracted. Pediatr Res 4:462, 1970

43. Bellanti JA, Cantz BE, Maybee DA, et al: Defective phagocytosis by newborn leucocytes: A defect similar to that in chronic granulomatous disease? Abstracted. Pediatr Res 3:376, 1969

44. Kretschmer RR, Papierniak CK, Stewardson-Krieger P, et al: Quantitative nitroblue tetrazolium reduction by normal newborn monocytes. J Pediatr 90:306–309, 1977

45. Das M, Klein W, Feig SA: Glycolytic metabolism of neonatal mononuclear cells. Pediatr Res 11:1026–1030, 1977

6
Humoral Mediators

Major advances have occurred in the recognition and characterization of the biologic interactions of mediators of the immune-inflammatory response. The mediators can conveniently be grouped into two major categories—plasma-derived factors and tissue-derived factors (Table 6-1). Of the plasma-derived factors, only those of the serum complement system have been extensively studied in the neonate.

COMPLEMENT

General Concepts

The serum complement system mediates a wide range of biologic activities. Several recent reviews have considered the general role of complement in host defenses.[1,2] Here, we will consider those aspects unique to the fetus and newborn.

Table 6-1
Mediators of Inflammation

	Major Groups	Major Mediators
Plasma factors	Complement system	C3a, C5a, C567, C-kinin
	Kinin system	Bradykinin, kallikrein
	Clotting system	Fibrinopeptides
Tissue factors	Amines	Histamine, 5-HT
	Acidic lipids	SRS-A, prostaglandins
	Lysomal components	Cationic proteins, acid proteases, neutral proteases
	Lymphocyte products	MIF, chemotactic factors, skin negative factors, LNPF
	Others	E.g., substance P

From Ryan GB: Beitr Pathd Bd 152:272–291, 1974.

Basic principles of complement function have been summarized by Johnston and Stroud:[1] (1) Complement consists of a system of interacting proteins (Table 6-2). Biologic functions derive from activation and interaction among these proteins. (2) The proteins interact in an orderly sequence, or "cascade," analogous to activation of the coagulation system. Once the first component has been activated, subsequent components are activated by the previous component or components in the sequence. (3) There are two recognized pathways of activation of complement (Fig. 6-1). In the *classical pathway,* the components interact in the sequence antigen–antibody–C142356789; in the *alternative or properdin pathway,* activation is in the order activator–(antibody)–properdin system–C356789. Although the precise nature of activation of these pathways in not fully understood, the concept of activation of complement at different sites by different mechanisms is important in establishing a broad biologic role for this system.

Table 6-2
Proteins of the Complement System

Units	Synonym	Molecular Weight	Serum Concentration (μg/ml)
Activation units			
C1q		400,000	200
C1r		168,000	
C1s	C1 esterase	79,000	120
C1t			
C4	β1E	240,000	400
C2		117,000	30
IF	C3NeF	150,000	Trace
Factor B	C3PA, GBG	100,000	225
Factor D	C3Pase, GBGase	25,000	Trace
Properdin		190,000	20
Properdin convertase		70,000	?
Functional units			
C3	β1C	180,000	1200
C5	β1F	185,000	75
C6		125,000	60
C7		120,000	60
C8		150,000	15
C9		79,000	Trace

From Spitzer RA: Pediatr Clin North Am 24:341–364, 1977.

Functional Activities of Complement

As a result of activation of complement, a number of biologic activities may be derived. These may involve (1) a cell membrane or antigen–antibody complex with which complement has interacted, or (2) biologically active principles released into the blood or other fluid compartments. Three types of biologic activity are derived from complement:

1. Cytotoxic reactions occur as a result of interaction of all components upon a particular cell surface or membrane. In the classical model of sheep cell hemolysis, for example, the end result of complement reaction upon the sensitized sheep

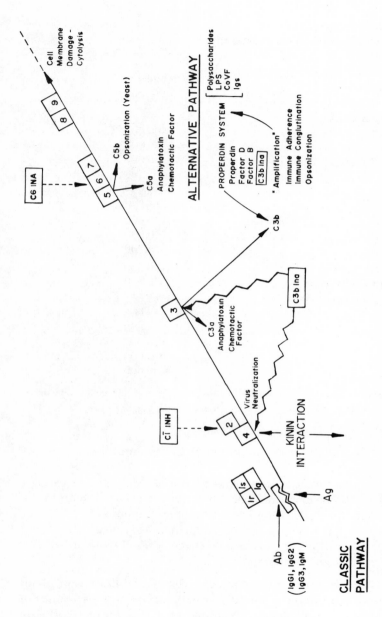

Fig. 6-1. Classic and alternative pathways of complement activation. (Modified from Miller ME: J Allergy Clin Immunol 51:45–56, 1973; and Johnston RB Jr, Stroud RM: J Pediatr 90:169–179, 1977.)

erythrocyte membrane is damage to the membrane, the result of which is an osmotic lysis secondary to the hole that has been "punched" in the membrane. Complement reaction can damage virtually any type of cell, lysis being but one example of such an effect.

2. A second type of complement-mediated biologic activity involves changes that occur upon the membrane involved in the complement reaction as the individual components react in sequence. For example, a pneumococcus that has reacted with antibody and has activated the complement sequence becomes far more readily phagocytized once the first four components have reacted. In other words, total reaction of the system may result in cytotoxic effects, but partial interaction may alter the entire antigen–antibody complex in such a way that phenomena such as opsonization and immune adherence take place.

3. The third type of biologic activity derives from low molecular weight "split products" of the native components which are released into the circulation upon activation of the parent molecule. Such materials possess potent activities as histamine releasers (anaphylatoxins) and in the attraction of leukocytes (chemotactic factors). The elaboration of such biologically active materials into the circulation has obvious potential in a wide range of clinical disorders of the inflammatory response. Table 6-3 provides examples of each type of activity.

Measurement of Complement

Hemolytic activity and immunochemical quantitation of individual components are the most commonly employed measurements of complement. Such measurements may fail to reflect *functional* abnormalities of complement proteins, however.[2,3] This is illustrated by the following study.[3]

Fresh whole blood from normal human volunteers was drawn into acid-citrate-dextrose (ACD) solution under usual blood-bank conditions and stored at 4°C. Each day, an aliquot was removed and studied for a number of complement-dependent activities. Two types of assays were performed: (1) quantitative and qualitative assays, including hemolytic activity, serum complement im-

Table 6-3
Examples of Functional Types of Complement Activity

	Components or Fragments	Functional Activity
1. Cytotoxic	C1~6 (? additional components)	Endotoxin inactivation
	C1~9	Lysis of viruses, virus-infected cells, tumor cells, mycoplasma, protozoa, spirochetes, and bacteria
2. Intermediate membrane alteration	C14, C1423	Virus neutralization
	C3b	Opsonization
	C3b, C3d	Enhanced induction of antibody formation
	C3b	Enhancement of antibody-dependent cellular cytotoxicity
	C3b	Stimulation of B-cell lymphokine production
	C5	Opsonization of fungi
3. Biologically active humoral mediators	C3a, C5a	"Anaphylatoxin" (capillary dilatation)
	C3a, C5a fragments, C567	Chemotaxis of PMNs, monocytes, eosinophils
	C3 cleavage product	Induction of granulocytosis

Modified from Johnston RB Jr, Stroud RA: J Pediatr 90:169–179, 1977.

mune adherence activity, and immunochemical conversion of C3 and C3 concentration (β_1C/β_1A), and (2) functional assays of opsonic activity toward baker's yeast and human erythrocytes and generation of chemotactic activity following incubation with antigen–antibody complexes. In the first group of assays, no losses of activity were detected over a 10-day period (Fig. 6-2). By usual standards, therefore, such material would be considered to possess "normal" complement activity. When opsonic and chemotactic activities of the same aliquots were observed, however, a different picture was seen (Fig. 6-3). Not only did all three

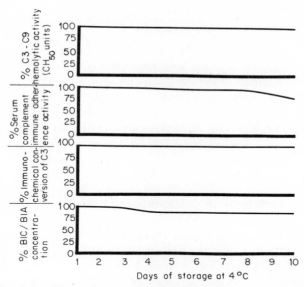

Fig. 6-2. Measurement of complement by hemolytic, immune adherence and immunochemical assays. (From Miller ME, Nilsson UR: Clin Immunol Immunopathal 2:246–255, 1974.)

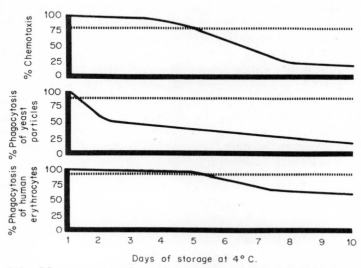

Fig. 6-3. Measurement of complement by opsonic and chemotactic assays. (From Miller ME, Nilsson UR: Clin Immunol Immunopathol 2:246-255, 1974.)

assays show a significant decline by the tenth day of storage, but the rate of decline was different for each activity studied, suggesting different functional complement requirements for each.

Such differences between quantitative and functional parameters of complement must be considered in the interpretation of published studies of complement in the fetus and newborn. The majority of studies have considered quantitations which, as illustrated above, may not reflect biologic activities.

Ontogeny of Complement in the Neonate

Three basic techniques have been utilized in studies of ontogeny of complement in human neonates:[4] (1) synthesis of individual components by isolated fetal tissues, usually by incorporation of radiolabeled markers into intact molecules; (2) demonstration of maternal–fetal discordance of genetic type where genetic polymorphisms exist, such as with C3 and C3PA; and (3) identification of a specific component in fetal or neonatal sera which the mother lacks as a result of a genetically determined deficiency, thus implying fetal synthesis of that component.

In man, such studies suggest that most complement components are synthesized early in fetal life. Synthesis of C3 in fetal tissues has been demonstrated by immunochemical techniques as early as 5.5 weeks of gestation,[5] therefore preceding that of immunoglobulins. Little or no placental transfer of maternal complement to the fetal circulation occurs.[2,4] C4 and C2 are apparently produced by macrophages, while C3, C5, C6, C9, and possibly C2 are synthesized in the liver. Synthesis of various complement components has been linked to the H-2 gene in mice and the HL-A system in man,[6] suggesting a possible role for complement as a recognition unit.

Complement In Neonates

HEMOLYTIC AND IMMUNOCHEMICAL MEASUREMENTS

A number of investigators have examined complement levels in term and/or premature infants. The results of these studies are summarized in Table 6-4. It is seen that many individual compo-

Table 6-4
Summary of Published Data
of Complement Levels in
Neonates (% Adult Levels)

C1q	75%
C3	56%
C4	55%
C5	60%
C3PA	50%
CH_{50}	50%

nents and total hemolytic activity are significantly decreased relative to adult values.

FUNCTIONAL MEASUREMENTS

Opsonic activity.   The importance of humoral factors, or "opsonins" in the enhancement of phagocytosis has been recognized since the turn of the century.[7] There are many opsonins in plasma, including antibodies and a variety of heat-stable and heat-labile proteins. The serum complement system plays an important role in opsonization of bacteria, and repeated data suggest deficiencies of complement-dependent opsonization in neonates.

Controversy exists in the selection of an appropriate assay system for the study of opsonization and phagocytosis. In particular, the type of particle being opsonized, the method of measurement of particle uptake, and the particle–phagocyte ratio are important variables.[8] Despite their differences, virtually all reported studies of opsonization by neonatal plasma or serum have demonstrated significant deficiencies relative to adult values.

Table 6-5 summarizes studies of neonatal phagocytosis. The earlier studies (group I) compared phagocytosis by whole blood of infants with that by whole blood of normal adults. Later studies (group II) separated plasma and cells, thereby more directly measuring opsonization. Although the general trend of these data indicate relatively decreased opsonization by neonatal sera, some inconsistencies remain.

Dossett and co-workers, for example, found opsonic activities of newborns less than those of maternal sera for *E. coli* and *S. marcescens* but similar for *S. aureus* and group B streptococcus.[9]

Table 6-5
Studies of Phagocytosis by Neonatal PMN

Group I—Whole Blood
   Tuniclifffe, 1910[21]
   Bracco, 1948[22]
   Matoth, 1952[23]
   Criscione, 1955[24]
   Arditi and Nigro, 1957[25]
   Sato, 1959[26]
   Miyamoto, 1965[27]

Group II—Separate Humoral and Cellular Components
   Gluck and Silverman, 1957[28]
   Cocchi and Marianelli, 1967[29]
   Miller, 1969[14]
   Forman and Stiehm, 1969[10]
   Coen et al., 1969[30]
   Park et al., 1969[31]
   Dossett et al., 1969[9]
   McCracken and Eichenwald, 1971[11]

Forman and Stiehm, however, found no opsonic deficiency of sera from term neonates against either *S. aureus* 502A or the same strain of *S. marcescens* used by Dosset and co-workers[10] (sera from 12 of 13 infants less than 1923 gm were, however, deficient in opsonic activities against both organisms). McCracken and Eichenwald studied the opsonic activity of neonatal sera for *S. aureus* 502A, *E. coli,* and *P. aeruginosa.*[11] At serum concentrations of 10 to 25 percent, opsonic activity varied with the birth weights of the infants. Infants weighing less than 3000 gm showed diminished opsonic activities for all three organisms. The observed opsonic deficiencies were considerably greater for gram-negative bacteria than for staphylococci.

Nature of the opsonic deficiencies.—Accumulating evidence suggests a primary role for complement in the opsonic deficiencies of neonatal plasma and serum, although the nature of this role and the number of components involved are not well characterized. Early inquiries into the problem focused upon the role of antibodies and their relationships to the recognized susceptibility of neonates to gram-negative organisms. In mice, Michael and Rosen demonstrated that IgM antibodies were a 1000-fold more efficient that IgG antibodies in bactericidal and opsonic activities against gram-negative organisms.[12] Subsequently, Gitlin and co-workers showed that bactericidal antibodies against *E. coli and S. typhosa* 0901 were poorly transferred across the placenta, despite the presence of adequate maternal serum titers against these organisms.[13] Less than 40 percent of sera from the infants contained bactericidal activities against *E. coli,* and only 20 percent had activity against *Salmonella.* In those cord sera that contained bactericidal activity against either of these organisms, antibodies were exclusively within the IgG class. When only maternal antibody activity was present, the antibodies were exclusively within the IgM class. It was therefore suggested that the susceptibility of newborns to gram-negative infections might be explained by a deficiency of placentally transferred IgM antibodies.

This deficiency, however, provides only a partial explanation for the opsonic deficiency or deficiencies of neonatal serum. In the yeast phagocytosis system, Miller found that the addition of purified IgM to neonatal serum failed to significantly enhance opsonic activity.[14] Dossett and co-workers found that the addition of complement or other heat-labile factors was necessary to significantly amplify opsonic activities of IgG and IgM.[9] Enhancing effects were far greater with IgM than with IgG. They concluded that while IgM antibodies are significant opsonins for *E. coli,* complement is necessary for the expression of full activity.

Forman and Stiehm studied opsonization in low-birth-weight (less than 1925 gm) infants.[10] In preliminary data on 6 infants, opsonic deficiencies improved in vivo following intramuscular injection of Cohn fraction II (largely IgG globulin) or in vitro following addition of IgG to the assay system. These results are intriguing in view of the presumed normal transfer of IgG from maternal to fetal circulations (Chapter 3).

McCracken and Eichenwald found a relationship between C3 concentrations and opsonic activity against *S. aureus* and *P. aeruginosa* but not against *E. coli.*[11] In yeast phagocytosis, Miller demonstrated a functional deficiency of the fifth component of complement (C5) in neonatal sera.[15]

Functional implications of alternative pathway deficiencies upon neonatal opsonization have not yet been reported.

Therapeutic considerations.—In the face of incomplete characterization of the opsonic deficiency or deficiencies of the neonate, it is not yet possible to establish definitive therapy. In summarizing the above studies, it appears that neonatal sera are deficient in opsonic activity for gram-negative bacteria, and, to a lesser extent, for *S. aureus*. Functional deficiencies tentatively identified include IgM, IgG, C3, and C5, each of which is contained in full activity in fresh plasma. Accordingly, several authors have suggested fresh plasma infusions in the management of neonatal septicemia.[9,15,16] Davis and co-workers observed increased opsonic activity toward *E. coli* in plasma of premature infants (1000–2000 gm) transfused with fresh adult blood.[16] Available data are not yet sufficient, however, to recommend the routine use of this approach in neonates, and controlled studies are necessary to establish the point.

Chemotactic activity. Miller studied generation of chemotactic activity from whole, fresh serum of term neonates incubated with gram-negative or gram-positive bacteria or antigen–antibody complexes.[17] Normal adult leukocytes were used as the responding cells. In the presence of standardized numbers of adult PMN, significantly less chemotactic activity was generated from neonatal than from adult serum for all three generating materials. Similar results have been reported by other investigators.[18] Although the nature of the chemotactic deficiency or deficiencies of neonatal sera has not been established, it seems likely that complement is involved.

OTHER MEDIATORS

Little discussion of factors other than complement is provided here, as there are few studies of their functional development in the neonate. Some data are available on the developmental status of coagulation factors in the newborn.[19] At birth, and increasingly over the first few days of life, profound decreases of vitamin-K-dependent factors may occur. These include prothrombin, factor VIII, factor IX, and factor X. Factor XI is also decreased. Hageman factor levels vary widely in neonates and may be depressed.[20] The functional implications of these deficiencies are unknown.

REFERENCES

1. Johnston RB Jr, Stroud RM: Complement and host defense against infection. J Pediatr 90:169–179, 1977
2. Spitzer RE: The complement system. Pediatr Clin North Am 24:341–364, 1977
3. Miller ME, Nilsson UR: A major role for the fifth component of complement (C5) in the opsonization of yeast particles. Partial dichotomy of functional and immunochemical measurement. Clin Immunol Immunopathol 2:246–255, 1974
4. Colten HR; Development of host defenses: The complement and properdin systems, in Cooper MD, Dayton DH (eds): Development of Host Defenses. New York, Raven Press, 1977, pp 165–173
5. Gitlin D, Biasucci A: Development of gamma-G, gamma-A, gamma-M, beta IC/beta 1A, Cl esterase inhibitor, ceruloplasmin, transferrin, hemopexin, haptoglobin, fibrinogen, plasminogen, alpha 1-antitrypsin, orosomucoid, beta-lipoprotein, alpha 2-macroglobulin, and prealbumin in the human conceptus. J Clin Invest 48:1422–1446, 1969
6. Wolski KP, Schmid FR, Mittal KK: Genetic linkage between the HL-A system and a deficiency of the second component (C2) of complement. Science 188:1020–1022, 1975
7. Metchnikoff E: Lectures on the Comparative Pathology of Inflammation. London, Kegan, Paul, Trench, Trubner and Company, 1893
8. Miller ME: Neutrophil function. Clin Immunol 3:427–437, 1976
9. Dossett JH, Williams RC Jr, Quie PG: Studies on interaction of bacteria, serum factors and polymorphonuclear leukocytes in mothers and newborns. Pediatrics 44:49–57, 1969
10. Forman ML, Stiehm ER: Impaired opsonic activity but normal phagocytosis in low-birth-weight infants. N Engl J Med 281:926–931, 1969
11. McCracken GH, Eichenwald HF: Leukocyte function and the development of opsonic and complement activity in the neonate. Am J Dis Child 121:120–126, 1971
12. Michael JG, Rosen FS: Association of "natural" antibodies to gram-negative bacteria with the gamma-1 macroglobulins. J Exp Med 118:619–626, 1963
13. Gitlin D, Rosen FS, Michael JG: Transient 19S gamma-globulin deficiency in the newborn infant and its significance. Pediatrics 31:197–208, 1963
14. Miller ME: Phagocytosis in the newborn infant: Humoral and cellular factors. J Pediatr 74:255–259, 1969
15. Miller ME: Demonstration and replacement of a functional defect of the fifth component of complement in newborn serum. A major tool

to the therapy of neonatal septicemia, abstracted. Pediatr Res 5:379–380, 1971

16. Davis AT, Blum PM, Quie PG: Studies on opsonic activity for *E. coli* in premature infants after blood transfusion, abstracted. Soc Pediatr Res, 1971, p 233

17. Miller ME: Chemotactic function in the human neonate: Humoral and cellular aspects. Pediatr Res 5:487–492, 1971

18. Pahwa S, Pahwa R, Grimes E, et al: Cellular and humoral components of monocyte and neutrophil chemotaxis in cord blood. Pediatr Res 11:677–680, 1977

19. Bleyer WA, Hakami N, Shepard TH: The development of hemostasis in the human fetus and newborn infant. J Pediatr 79:838–853, 1971

20. Kurkcuoglu M, McElfresh AE: The Hageman factor. Determination of the concentration during the neonatal period and presentation of a case of Hageman factor deficiency. J Pediatr 57:61–65, 1960

21. Tunicliffe R: Observations on anti-infectious power of blood of infants. J Infect Dis 7:698–707, 1910

22. Bracco G: Potere fagocitari: Del sangoe placentare fetali. G Batteriol Immunol 38:449–456, 1948

23. Matoth Y: Phagocytic and ameboid activities of the leukocytes in the newborn infant. Pediatrics 9:748–754, 1952

24. Criscione C: Compartamento dell immunita naturale aspecifica nel prematuro confrontata con quella dei nati a termine a maturi. Aggiorn Pediatr 6:323, 1955

25. Arditi E, Nigro N: II potere fagocitario del sangue nell'immaturo. G Mal Infett 8:581–583, 1957

26. Sato T: The phagocytosis of India ink by leukocytes in premature infants. Niigata Med J 73:24–31, 1959

27. Miyamoto K: Phagocytic activity of leucocytes in premature infants. I. Comparison of the phagocytic activity of leucocytes between premature infants and full term infants. Hiroshima J Med Sci 14:9–17, 1965

28. Gluck L, Silverman WA: Phagocytosis in premature infants. Pediatrics 20:951–957, 1957

29. Cocchi P, Marianelli L: Phagocytosis and intracellular killing of Pseudomonas aeruginosa in premature infants. Helv Paediat Acta 22:110–118, 1967

30. Coen R, Grush O, Kauder E: Studies of bactericidal activity and metabolism of the leukocyte in full-term neonates. J Pediatr 75:400–406, 1969

31. Park BH, Holmes B, Good RA: Metabolic activities in leukocytes of newborn infants. J Pediatr 76:237–241, 1970

7
Clinical Disorders of Host Defense

We consider here the clinical disorders of immune or inflammatory deficiency in the neonate. For several reasons, specific diagnoses of deficient host defenses are uniquely difficult to establish during this period of life. First, as detailed in the preceding chapters, many neonatal host defenses are developmentally immature. What is abnormal for the newborn, therefore, often becomes a matter of subjective judgment. Second, placentally transferred maternal cells and/or humoral factors may influence the various in vitro assays of immune inflammatory function. A definitive diagnosis of a specific defect of host defenses must therefore sometimes be delayed until a later age.

DISORDERS OF THE T-CELL SYSTEM

Clinical Findings

GENERAL

Immunodeficiencies involving T-cell system in neonates often present a typical general clinical picture. Among the findings common to this group of disorders are (1) marked wasting, debilitation, or "runted" appearance; (2) rashes, particularly generalized maculopapular rashes with alopecia, which may be noted in graft-versus-host reactions; (3) perianal or perioral candidiasis, especially if associated with diarrhea or, more commonly, steatorrhea; (4) deficient lymphoid tissue, especially in the presence of a regional infection; (5) persistent infection, often of a mixed nature including viral, bacterial, fungal and protozoal organisms.

SPECIFIC

In addition to the above general clinical features, many disorders of the T-cell system have characteristic features (Table 7-1). Syndromes included in this category are the DiGeorge syndrome, chronic mucocutaneous candidiasis, Nezelof's syndrome, Wiskott-Aldrich syndrome, immunodeficiency with enzyme deficiency, and severe combined immunodeficiency disease.

The *DiGeorge syndrome* results from abnormal embryologic development of the third and fourth pharyngeal pouches at approximately 12 weeks of gestation.[1] The thymus and parathyroid glands develop from epithelial evaginations of these structures at approximately 6 to 8 weeks of gestation, and caudal migration of the thymus occurs at 12 weeks. At the same time, the philtrum of the lip, ear tubercle, and aortic arch structures are differentiated. The DiGeorge syndrome thus represents a group of disorders involving the thymus, the parathyroids, and the cardiovascular and facial structures. Clinical findings frequently present shortly after birth. The usual presenting signs involve cardiovascular abnormalities and/or hypoparathyroidism—i.e., tetany—with immunologic complications usually occurring later. The combination of abnormal facies, congenital heart disease, and recalcitrant

Table 7-1
Clinical Features of T-Cell and Partial T-B Cell
Immunodeficiency Disorders

Clinical Features	Disorders
Immunologic	
Recurrent viral infection	DiGeorge, chronic candidiasis, and T-B cell deficiency
Fungal and protozoal infection	DiGeorge, chronic candidiasis, and T-B cell deficiency
Recurrent bacterial infection	DiGeorge and T-B cell immuno-deficiency
Dermatologic	
Eczema	Wiskott-Aldrich, T-B cell immunodeficiency
Telangiectasia	Ataxia-telangiectasia
Petechiae	Wiskott-Aldrich
Endocrinologic	
Hypoparathyroidism (congenital)	DiGeorge
Hypoparathyroidism (acquired)	Chronic candidiasis
Hypothyroidism, Addison's, diabetes	Chronic candidiasis
Gonadal dysgenesis	Chronic candidiasis and ataxia-telangiectasia
Neurologic	
Ataxia	Ataxia-telangiectasia
Hematologic	
Thrombocytopenia	Wiskott-Aldrich
Anemia (pernicious)	Chronic candidiasis
Anemia (Coombs' +)	Wiskott-Aldrich
Skeletal	
Short-limbed dwarfism	Short-limbed dwarfism with immunodeficiency
Bony abnormalities	Immunodeficiency with adenosine deaminase deficiency
Biochemical	
Adenosine deaminase deficiency	Immunodeficiency with adenosine deaminase deficiency
Nucleoside phosphorylase deficiency	Immunodeficiency with nucleoside phosphorylase deficiency

From Ammann AJ: Pediatr Clin North Am 24:293–311, 1977.

hypoparathyroidism in an infant should arouse suspicion of Di-George syndrome. Features of the abnormal facies may include hypertelorism, notched ear pinnae, micrognathia, antimongoloid slant of the eyes, fish-shaped mouth, and low set ears. Bifid uvula, urinary tract abnormallties, and esophageal atresia have also been described.

Chronic mucocutaneous candidiasis lies at the opposite end of the spectrum of relatively "pure" T-cell disorders.[2] In the Di-George syndrome, T-cell function is virtually absent, while patients with chronic mucocutaneous candidiasis usually have only minor deficiencies of T-cell activities. Chronic candidiasis probably also represents a heterogeneous group of disorders. The major clinical presentation consists of chronic candidal infection of the skin and mucous membranes and/or nails. In some patients, the candidiasis occurs in association with idiopathic endocrinopathy, including (in order of frequency) hypoparathyroidism, Addison's disease, hypothyroidism, and/or diabetes. On occasion, pernicious anemia and gonadal dysgenesis also occur. Multiple endocrinopathy in association with chronic candidiasis may represent generalized autoimmune disorder(s) in which the thymus and other endocrine glands are involved. The chronic candidiasis syndromes rarely present during the neonatal period.

Nezelof's syndrome includes disorders of deficient T-cell function with variable B-cell function. Disorders classified in this category[3] are undoubtedly diverse in etiology. Chronic otitis media and sinusitis often occur, and infections are likely to be multiple, including viral, bacterial, fungal, and protozoal organisms. In general, patients with Nezelof's syndrome may experience a somewhat milder clinical course than those with severe combined immunodeficiency. The diagnosis of Nezelof's syndrome is difficult to establish during the neonatal period owing to the highly variable clinical course and the difficulty of definitive laboratory diagnosis of B- and T-cell function (see below) during this period of life.

Severe combined immunodeficiency disease (SCID) is the most severe and, along with the DiGeorge syndrome, the most clinically characteristic form of immunodeficiency occurring during the neonatal period. Onset of symptoms frequently occurs during the first month of life. Without treatment, death is inevitable by 1 to 2 years of age. Although initially regarded as a defect in stem cell immunity, it is now apparent that SCID encompasses multiple etiologies, ranging from deficiencies of thymic maturation to primary enzyme abnormalities. Two major genetic patterns of inheritance occur—an X-linked recessive form (originally termed X-linked lymphopenic agammaglobulinemia) and an autosomal recessive form (originally termed Swiss type or autosomal recessive lymphopenic agammaglobulinemia).[4,5] Clinical findings in SCID include most of the general features listed above. Occasional patients present with short-limbed dwarfism, characterized by shortened extremities, redundant skinfolds, and metaphyseal dysotosis of long bones. SCID and short-limbed dwarfism are part of a spectrum of immunodeficiency with short-limbed dwarfism which may involve only T-cell or B-cell deficiency. Another group of such patients present with cartilage-hair hypoplasia and/or neutropenia along with variable immunodeficiency and short-limbed dwarfism.

Graft-versus-host (GVH) reactions are frequently encountered in patients with SCID. Such reactions may originate from maternal cells transferred to the fetus during gestation[6] or at delivery or from the postnatal transfusion of blood products that contain viable lymphocytes. Since patients with SCID are often critically ill, they not uncommonly receive blood transfusions for supportive care. If one suspects the possibility of SCID or other form of T-cell deficiency, it is extremely important that blood products be administered only if absolutely necessary, and then with extreme care to eliminate viable lymphocytes. Such measures include irradiation (3000–4000 R) or freezing. The clinical signs of GVH reactions include a maculopapular rash (sometimes desquamating), jaundice, diarrhea, hepatosplenomegaly, anemia, thrombocytopenia, generalized edema, tachypnea, cardiac arrhythmias, hypertension, and general irritability.[6] More severe forms of GVH reaction may also cause a picture similar to toxic epidermal necrolysis or acrodermatitis enteropathica.

Two forms of *immunodeficiency with enzyme deficiency* have been described. Adenosine deaminase (ADA) deficiency has been associated with both T- and B-cell deficiency, while nucleoside phosphorylase deficiency has been associated with T-cell deficiency.[2,7] Both deficiencies follow an autosomal recessive pattern of inheritance. The mechanism or mechanisms by which these deficiencies relate to immunodeficiency are speculative.[2] Patients with ADA deficiency and SCID are clinically indistinguishable from those with other forms of SCID except that the former may have characteristic radiographic findings including concavity and flaring of the anterior ribs, abnormal contour and articulation of the posterior ribs and transverse processes, thick growth arrest lines, an abnormal bony pelvis, and platyspondylisis. Patients with ADA deficiency and SCID may present during the neonatal period, but those wtih nucleoside phosphorylase deficiency and immunodeficiency (usually absent T-cell and normal B-cell immunity) often remain asymptomatic until 6 to 12 months of age.

Wiskott-Aldrich syndrome is a sex-linked recessive disorder that involves immunodeficiency, thrombocytopenia, eczema, and recurrent infections. Symptoms that often occur at or around birth are related to the thrombocytopenia and may present bleeding from the gastrointestinal tract or circumcision site. The nature of the immunologic defects in this syndrome is poorly understood.[8,9] Variable T- and B-cell abnormalities may be absent at birth and occur with increasing age. One hypothesis suggests that the primary etiology of Wiskott-Aldrich syndrome is a defect in macrophage processing of polysaccharide antigens. This might explain the undue susceptibility of afflicted children to such infections as *H. influenzae, Pneumococcus,* and *E. coli.* The combination of eczema, thrombocytopenia, and bleeding in a male infant suggests a diagnosis of Wiskott-Aldrich syndrome. T- and B-cell abnormalities are variable, but B-cell deficiencies are more consistently observed. Isohemagglutinins may be low to absent, and a pattern of normal to elevated IgG, decreased IgM, and elevated IgA and IgE is frequently seen.

Diagnosis of T Cell Disorders

GENERAL PARAMETERS

Lymphoid tissue.   Primary disorders of the T-cell system are usually associated with decreased lymphoid mass. This can usually be suspected clinically by the absence of tonsils or palpable lymph nodes. Confirmatory radiologic diagnosis can be obtained by a lateral neck film. Patients with Nezelof's syndrome provide an occasional exception to this rule and may actually have enlarged lymph nodes.

Thymic tissue.   Absence of thymic shadow on P-A and lateral chest film is usually found in congenital T-cell deficiency states.

Esophagitis.   Monilial esophagitis produces a family characteristic radiographic pattern that can often be detected with a barium swallow. If other potential causes of this picture, such as lye ingestion, can be ruled out, this provides a very helpful diagnostic aid.[10]

Blood picture.   Although not diagnostic, a number of peripheral blood findings are supportive of a diagnosis of T-cell deficiency. These include: (1) Lymphopenia—when present, this is helpful. Normal lymphocyte counts are sometimes present, however, and do *not* rule out a diagnosis of primary T-cell deficiency.[4] (2) Eosinophilia and monocytosis—these are frequently observed in patients with severe combined immune deficiency. A unique characteristic is the frequent day-to-day variability. Eosinophil counts, for example, may be as high as 45 to 50 percent one day, and monocytes may rise to the same levels the next day with frequent interchange of values. The eosinophils may show abnormal morphology.[11] (3) Thrombocytopenia—when present, this may suggest Wiskott-Aldrich syndrome, although it may also be observed in septicemia and GVH reactions. (4) Anemia—this is frequently observed but may not be apparent during the neonatal period. (5) Neutropenia—this is frequently observed in T-cell deficiency states and may reflect septicemia or be associated with cartilage-hair hypoplasia and short-limbed dwarfism. (Primary disorders of the neutrophil are discussed later in this chapter.) (6) "Plasmacytoid lymphocytes" and erythrophagocytosis—if seen on smear, these may suggest GVH disease.[12,13]

Serum electrolytes.   Low serum calcium levels in association with elevated serum phosphorous levels suggest hypoparathyroidism and may be seen in the DiGeorge syndrome. Patients with nucleoside phosphorylase deficiency are unable to form uric acid and, consequently, may have low levels of serum and/or urine uric acid.

Enzyme assays. Adenosine deaminase deficiency may be diagnosed by measurement of enzyme activity in a number of tissues, including erythrocytes, leukocytes, and cultured amniotic fluid cells. Diagnosis is most easily made by assaying erythrocytes.

IMMUNOLOGIC ASSAYS

An ever-increasing number of measurements for the assay of T-cell function are now available (Chapter 2). Although it is probable that accurate laboratory diagnosis of T-cell disorders will ultimately be available, currently utilized techniques still fail to provide clear-cut diagnoses. Available tests fall into two basic categories—screening and diagnostic.[14] For screening purposes, a total lymphocyte count is helpful when low, but if the count is normal this test does not provide much aid in diagnosis (see above). Delayed hypersensitivity skin tests are a second commonly employed screening technique for T-cell deficiencies. Interpretation of such data in the neonate is so difficult, however, that their diagnostic value is marginal (Chapter 4). Diagnostic test are of two types—quantitative and functional. Currently utilized quantitative assays include the E (erythrocyte) rosette technique, in which human T cells bind to sheep erythrocytes to form rosettes[15-17] and indirect immunofluorescence using antisera with specificity against T-cell surface antigenic markers. Available data in newborns differ with these assays, depending upon whether cord blood or peripheral venous blood is utilized. Further, the number of T cells detected by these two methods may differ. It is not clear whether this reflects differences in sensitivity between the two assays or the identification of separate markers. Detection of T-cell subsets is still in a primitive stage. Although separate markers for helper and suppressor T cells have been described,[18] their clinical accuracy, particularly in the neonate, remains to be demonstrated. Functional properties of T cells can be evaluated by three types of assay: in vitro response to mitogens (PHA), antigens, or allogeneic cells (mixed lymphocyte culture); effector cell responses, including cell-mediated and

during the early months of life. In the summary that follows, it should therefore be borne in mind that diagnostic suspicion may not be confirmed until the patient is well beyond the neonatal period.

Disorders of Cell Movement.   Several mechanisms of phagocyte movement, directed and random, are recognized (Chapter 5). Disorders of movement may be partially characterized by defining the functional status of each type of movement.

This subject has been extensively reviewed.[40,41] Four basic types of defect exist: (1) intrinsic selective defects in which a primary abnormality of cell function results in deficiencies solely of movement; (2) intrinsic combined defects in which primary cellular defects result in abnormalities of movement and at least one other phagocyte function, such as phagocytosis or bactericidal activity; (3) defects of phagocyte movement due to circulating inhibitors that may act directly upon the cell or upon a chemotactic factor; and (4) defects resulting from abnormal production of chemotactic factors as, for example, in primary disorders of the complement system (see below). Tables 7-2 to 7-4 list some examples of movement disorders in each of these categories. With the increased recognition of disorders of PMN movement, the relationships between in vitro and in vivo measurements of PMN movement have become increasingly complex. In early descriptions of abnormal PMN movement, such as the "lazy leukocyte syndrome," a clear correlation between clinical and laboratory observations was evident. These patients suffered recurrent low-grade infections, were neutropenic, and failed to generate inflammatory cells normally in vivo by the skin-window technique.[42] PMN from these patients studied in vitro showed abnormal movement in both Boyden chamber and capillary tube assays. As indicated in Table 7-5, however, no single parameter can be considered characteristic of all disorders of PMN movement. For example, skin-window response and even peripheral PMN counts may be normal in patients with obvious in vitro defects of PMN movement. Recurrent low-grade infections, particularly of skin, respiratory tract, gingivae, and oral cavity are among the more common presenting clinical signs in patients

Table 7-2
Intrinsic Disorders of Phagocyte Movement*

	Directed Movement	Random Movement	Phagocytosis	Bactericidal Activity
1. *Intrinsic selective movements*				
Lazy leukocyte syndrome	→	→	N	N
Familial chemotactic defect	→	N	N	N
Candidiasis with decreased cell-mediated immunity	→	N →	N	N
Postdialysis neutropenia	± →	→	N	N
2. *Combined intrinsic defects*				
Chediak-Higashi syndrome	→	→ →	N	→ |
Defective actin polymerization	→	→	± →	
Neonatal leukocytes	→	N	±	± N

N = Normal.
*Reviewed in refs. 40 and 41.

Table 7-3
Disorders of Phagocyte Movement Secondary
to Circulating Inhibitors*

1. *Site of inhibition directly upon cell*
   Deficient monocyte chemotaxis in Wiskott-Aldrich syndrome
   Rheumatoid arthritis
   Serum inhibitor in child with recurrent infections
2. *Site of inhibition upon chemotactic factors*
   Hodgkin's disease
   Cirrhosis
   Glomerulonephritis

*Reviewed in refs. 40 and 41.

with PMN movement defects. Such infections occurring in association with neutropenia and/or absence of pus or decreased inflammatory response suggest such an abnormality.

Disorders of phagocytosis. No isolated defects of intrinsic PMN phagocytosis have yet been described. Boxer and coworkers, however, described an infant with pyogenic infections from birth who had nonmotile neutrophils that were deficient in chemotaxis and phagocytosis.[43] Actin isolated from the infant's PMN was normal in amount but failed to polymerize under conditions that fully polymerized actin in normal neutrophils.

Disorders of bactericidal activity. Interest in disorders of bactericidal activity of PMN derives largely from the recognition

Table 7-4
Disorders of Phagocyte Movement
Secondary to Defective Production
of Chemotactic Activities*

Disorders of complement
Disorders of kinin generation
Disorders of cellular-derived chemotactic factors

*Reviewed in refs. 40 and 41.

Table 7-5

In Vitro and In Vivo Correlates of PMN Movement Defect

Defect	PMN Count	PMN Migration*	Chemotaxis	Capillary Tube Migration	Epinephrine-Endotoxin Response
Chediak-Higashi	Diminished	Diminished or Normal	Diminished	Normal	Diminished
Lazy leukocyte syndrome	Diminished	Diminished	Diminished	Diminished	Diminished
Neonate	Moderately Diminished	Very Moderately Diminished	Diminished	Moderately Diminished	—
Diabetes	Normal	Moderately Diminished	Diminished	Normal	Normal
Familial chemotactic defect	Normal	Normal	Diminished	Normal	Normal
Rheumatoid arthritis	Variable	—	Diminished	—	—
Candidiasis with decreased cell-mediated activity		Moderately Diminished	Diminished	Normal	Normal
Dialysis with dow membrane	Decreased Throughout	—	Moderately Diminished	Totally Absent	—

*Skin-window (Rebuck) technique.
From Miller ME: Semin Hematol 12:59–82, 1975.

of chronic granulomatous disease (CGD) as a basic defect of phagocyte killing.[44] The syndrome of CGD consists of recurrent, suppurative infections of the skin, reticuloendothelial organs and lungs in association with inability of patient's phagocytes to kill catalase-positive, non-hydrogen-peroxide-producing bacteria such as staphylococci and enteric organisms. Catalase-negative, peroxide-producing organisms such as *H. influenzae,* streptococci, and pneumococci are relatively infrequent infecting organisms in CGD.

Onset of symptoms usually occurs within the first year of life, although in some patients initial infections have occurred as late as 12 years of age. Common clinical findings include suppurative lymphadenopathy, pneumonitis, dermatitis, hepatomegaly, and splenomegaly.

Two distinct genetic patterns of inheritance of CGD occur—X-linked and autosomal recessive. Several other varieties of the syndrome have been proposed but await complete characterization of the molecular defect(s) in CGD for confirmation.

Diagnosis of CGD is suggested by defective reduction of nitro-blue-tetrazolium (NBT) by patient's PMN during phagocytosis. Confirmation, however, requires demonstration of defective intracellular killing of ingested non-hydrogen-peroxide-producing organisms by patient's PMN.

Management of children with CGD remains nonspecific. The use of prophylactic or broad-spectrum antibiotics is controversial, and antimicrobial therapy should, therefore, be as specific as possible.

Several other causes for deficient PMN bactericidal activity have been proposed, including leukocyte glucose 6-phosphate dehydrogenase (G6PD) deficiency[45] and glutathione deficiency.[46] The former simulates the abnormality in CGD through defective production of hydrogen peroxide. In the latter, diminished capacity to detoxify hydrogen perioxide has been observed. Oliver and co-workers have suggested that the excess hydrogen peroxide may impair leukocyte functions through the damage of microtubules.[47]

The clinical spectrum of these disorders, particularly as they occur in the neonate, is unknown.

Disorders of Monocytes

It is unclear whether isolated deficiencies of only PMN or MNL function exist (Chapter 5).

Clinical and Laboratory Evaluation of Phagocyte Disorders

In general, patients with defective phagocyte function exhibit some abnormality of inflammation. For example, degree of fever or clinical toxicity may be disproportionate to that observed in normal patients with similar infections. When abscess formation occurs, it may be deficient in one or more basic parameters—pain, heat, erythema, or swelling. Unfortunately, the same is true of the normal neonatal inflammatory response, so that subtle abnormalities may not be recognized until later in life.

The in vitro evaluation of phagocyte functions should include at least one assay for *each* function being tested. Assays that measure "phagocytic killing," for example, may not be critical or sensitive enough to identify the precise type of functional PMN defect. Tables 7-6 and 7-7 list some of the commonly employed assays of phagocyte function.

Table 7-6
In Vivo Assays of Phagocyte Function

Assay	Comments
Inflammatory cycle	General screen—may not be abnormal in all cases of movement defects
Epinephrine response	Test marginating pool of PMNs
Hydrocortisone response	Test of marrow pool of PMNs. Less toxicity then endotoxin stimulation
Peripheral PMN count	May not always reflect functional PMN defect

Table 7-7
In Vitro Assays of Phagocyte Function

Function	Assays
Bactericidal activity	1. Direct killing by phagocyte—specific but technically cumbersome
	2. NBT reduction—good screen but must be confirmed by direct killing assay
Phagocytosis	1. Direct particle ingestion—specific but somewhat cumbersome.
	2. Metabolic assays—less specific but may lend better to large-scale studies
Movement	1. Boyden chamber assay and agarose assay—measure directed migration
	2. Capillary tube assay—measures undirected migration. Assays above may also be modified to measure undirected migration
	3. Elastimetry—measures deformability of cell

DISORDERS OF MEDIATORS

Disorders of Complement

Four basic types of abnormalities affecting the complement system are recognized[48,49]: (1) primary deficiencies of individual components of the classical or alternative pathways; (2) primary deficiencies of naturally occurring inhibitors of classical or alternative pathways; (3) functional, rather than quantitative, abnormalities of complement components or inhibitors (only classical pathway examples at present); and (4) complement deficiencies secondary to acquired inactivators of native components or their by-products. Examples of disorders occurring within each category are summarized in Tables 7-8 through 7-11.

Table 7-8
Primary Disorders of
Complement Components

Deficient Component*	
C1q	C5
C1r	C6
C4	C7
C2	C8
C3	C3PA

*Reviewed in ref. 48.

Table 7-9
Disorders of Naturally Occurring
Complement Inhibitors*

C1 esterase inhibitor (hereditary angioedema)

C3b inactivator

Table 7-10
Functional Abnormalities of
Complement Components

C1 esterase inhibitor 48, 49 ($\sim$ 10% of cases)

C5 dysfunction 50–53 (Leiner's syndrome)

Table 7-11
Inactivator Deficiencies
of Complement*

Hypercatabolism of C3 with nephritic factor

Hypercatabolism of C3 without nephritic factor

? Thermal injury

? Malnutrition

*Reviewed in refs. 48 and 49.

While any of these deficiencies can theoretically occur during the neonatal period, only C5 dysfunction (Leiner's disease) is likely to present a major diagnostic consideration.

C5 DYSFUNCTION (LEINER'S DISEASE)

In 1908, Leiner[50] published his observations on a series of infants who had a combination of symptoms consisting of a generalized erythroderma, frequent loose stools, and failure to thrive. Onset was generally under the age of 1 month, and duration of the illness varied from several weeks to several months. Fifteen of the original series of 43 infants (1902 to 1907) and 3 of the 14 infants in a later series (1907 to 1911) died. In a later dissertation, Leiner stressed the specificity of the condition, pointing in particular to the persistent severe gastrointestinal symptoms as the differentiating factor.

The dermatosis was described as universal erythema and loosening of the epidermis with scale and crust formation. The changes about the scalp and face resembled those of seborrheic dermatitis but did not always progress to the extreme crusting of seborrheic eczema. In the intertriginous areas, the lesions were more exudative and tended to accumulate greasy debris.

Leiner considered the presence of severe intestinal disturbance as pathognomonic for this disease. The intestinal manifestations consisted of frequent, loose, greenish, mucoid stools and occasionally vomiting, which might be projectile. The dermatologic and intestinal symptoms appeared to be interdependent; deterioration in one system let to worsening of the other, and vice versa. Failure to gain weight or actual loss of weight was always a consequence of the illness.

In Leiner's original series, there were twins who contracted the condition concurrently at 6 weeks of age and who recovered after 2 months. In another family, 2 infants, sequential in family order, contracted the condition at age 6 weeks and each died after an illness of several weeks. Thus, there is evidence among the very first cases for the possible presence of a genetic defect.

Subsequently, several children with a plasma-associated defect of phagocytosis were described[51,52] who presented with diarrhea, generalized seborrheiclike dermatitis, recurrent infections, and failure to thrive. In both families, a deficiency of opsonic activity of the fifth component of serum complement (C5) was demonstrated. The institution of treatment in each patient with infusions of fresh plasma resulted in dramatic clinical improvement. The similarities of these children to those described by Leiner were striking.

The initial experience with Leiner's patients and the more recently described infants with C5 dysfunction establish the existence of a treatable clinical entity of importance to the pediatrician. The syndrome is characterized by severe seborrheiclike dermatitis, intractable diarrhea, recurrent infections (mainly with gram-negative bacilli), and marked dystrophy. A diagnosis of seborrheic dermatitis, no matter how severe, is not in itself enough to establish a diagnosis of Leiner's disease.

Diagnosis is established by the demonstration of deficient opsonic activity of the patient's serum or plasma. Latex, erythrocytes, or pneumococci are not satisfactory particles for this assay.[52] The dysfunction of C5 is detected only by an assay that measures biologic activity of the protein in opsonization. Quantitative levels of C5 in these families, as measured by standard immunochemical techniques, are within normal limits. Adequate therapy includes infusion of material containing opsonically active C5; fresh plasma or blood is satisfactory, whereas refrigerated plasma or blood over 24 hours of age is not. It is hoped that a semipure preparation of C5 will eventually replace the need to utilize whole blood or plasma transfusions in the treatment of these patients.

An additional point of importance in Leiner's reports was his observation that the illness was limited almost exclusively to breast-fed infants. He noted that ". . . this dermatitis, about which I am reporting, represents a special type for itself, and it is of the greatest importance to be able to recognise it, for with few exceptions, it only attacks children at the breast. This disease, far from being harmless, very often is even extremely dangerous for the infants, and death from this form of dermatitis is not at all infrequent."[50] He observed clinical improvement upon placing such infants on bovine milk. Recent evidence of opsonic activity of milks supports these observations.[53]

Other Mediators

As discussed in the previous chapter, little is known of the functional implications of quantitative deficiencies in neonates of other mediators, such as those of the coagulation system.

REFERENCES

1. DiGeorge AM: Congenital absence of the thymus and its immunologic consequences: Concurrence with congenital hypoparathyroidism. Birth Defects 4:116–123, 1968
2. Ammann AJ: T cell and T-B cell immunodeficiency disorders. Pediatr Clin North Am 24:293–311, 1977
3. Lawlor GJ Jr, Ammann AJ, Wright WC: The syndrome of cellular immunodeficiencies with immunoglobulins. J Pediatr 84:183–192, 1974
4. Miller ME, Schieken RM: Thymic dysplasia. A separable entity from "Swiss agammaglobulinemia." Characterization of a distinct clinical entity. Am J Med Sci 253:741–750, 1967
5. Hitzig WH: Congenital thymic and lymphocytic deficiency disorders, in Steihm ER, Fulginit VA (eds): Immunologic Disorders in Infants and Children. Philadelphia, Saunders, 1973, pp 215–235
6. Buckley RH: Immunoreconstitution. Pediatr Clin North Am 24:313–328, 1977
7. Giblett ER, Anderson JE, Cohen F, et al: Adenosine deaminase deficiency in two patients with severely impaired cellular immunity. Lancet 2:1067–1069, 1972
8. Blaese RM, Strober W, Waldmann TA: Immunodeficiency in the Wiskott-Aldrich syndrome. Birth Defects 11:250–254, 1975
9. Cooper MD, Chase HP, Lowmann JT, et al: Immunologic defects in patients with Wiskott-Aldrich syndrome. Birth Defects 4:378–387, 1968
10. Borns PA: Personal communication.
11. Miller ME, Hummeler K: Thymic dysplasia ("Swiss agammaglobulinemia"). II. Morphologic and functional observations. J Pediatr 70:737–744, 1967
12. Miller ME: Thymic dysplasia ("Swiss agammaglobulinemia"). I. Graft versus host reaction following bone marrow transfusion. J Pediatr 70:730–736, 1967

13. Buckley RH: Replacement therapy in immunodeficiency, in Thompson RA (ed): Recent Advances in Clinical Immunology I. London, Churchill Livingston, 1978, (in press)

14. Wara DW: Laboratory diagnosis of immunodeficiency disease. Pediatr Clin North Am 24:329–339, 1977

15. Froland SS: Binding of sheep erythrocytes to human lymphocytes. A probable marker of T lymphocytes. Scand J Immunol 1:269–280, 1972

16. Greaves MF, Brown G: Purification of human T and B lymphocytes. J Immunol 112:420–423, 1974

17. Jondal M, Holm G, Wigzell H: Surface markers on human T and B lymphocytes. J Exp Med 136:207–215, 1972

18. Gupta S, Schwarta SA, Safai B, et al: Immunoregulatory T cell subpopulations in lymphoproliferative disorders. Clin Res 25:359A, 1977

19. Buckley RH: Transplantation, in Stiehm ER, Fulginiti VA (eds): Immunologic Disorders in Infants and Children. Philadelphia, Saunders, 1973, pp 591–623

20. Goldman AS, Goldblum RM: Primary deficiencies in humoral immunity. Pediatr Clin North Am 24:277–291, 1977

21. Miller ME, Stiehm ER: Phagocytic, opsonic, and immunoglobulin studies in newborns. Calif Med 119:43–63, 1973

22. Hodes HL: Should the premature infant receive gamma-globulin? Pediatrics 32:1–3, 1963

23. Amer J, Ott E, Ibbott FA, et al: The effect of monthly gamma-globulin administration on morbidity and mortality from infection in premature infants during the first year of life. Pediatrics 32:4–9, 1963

24. Hobbs JR, Davis JA: Serum gamma-G-globulin levels and gestational age in premature babies. Lancet 1:757–759, 1967

25. Bridges RA, Condie RM, Zak SJ, et al: The morphologic basis of antibody formation development during the neonatal period. J Lab Clin Med 53:331–357, 1959

26. Holland NH, Holland P: Immunological maturation in an infant of an agammaglobulinemic mother. Lancet 2:1152–1155, 1966

27. Lalezari P, Nussbaum M, Gelman S, et al: Neonatal neutropenia due to maternal isoimmunization. Blood 15:236–243, 1960

28. Boxer LA: Immunologic function and leukocyte disorders in newborn infants. Clin Hematol, Feb 1978, (in press)

29. Lalezari P, Radel E: Neutrophil-specific antigens: Immunology and clinical significance. Semin Hematol 11:281–290, 1974

30. Boxer LA, Yokoyama M, Lalezari P: Isoimmune neonatal neutropenia. J. Pediatr 80:783–787, 1972

31. Boxer LA, Stossel TP: Effects of antineutrophil antibodies in vitro. Quantitative studies. J Clin Invest 53:1534–1545, 1974

32. Miller ME and Boxer LA: Cell elastimetry in the detection of immune neutropenia—demonstration of a membrane perturbation, abstracted. Pediatr Res, 11:477, 1977

33. Adner MM, Fisch GR, Starobin SG, et al: Use of "compatible" platelet transfusions in treatment of genital isoimmune neonatal thrombocytopenic purpura. N Engl J Med 280:244–247, 1969

34. Pincus SH, Boxer LA, Stossel TP: Chronic neutropenia in childhood. Am J Med 61:849–861, 1976

35. Miller ME: Cell elastimetry in the characterization of normal and abnormal PMN movement, in Gallin JI, Quie PG (eds): Leukocyte Chemotaxis. New York, Raven Press, 1978, pp.379–387

36. Kostmann R: Infantile genetic agranulocytosis. Acta Pediatr Scand 64:362–368, 1975

37. Kostmann R: Infantile genetic agranulocytosis. Acta Pediatr Scand 45 (Suppl 105): 1–78, 1956

38. L'Esperance P, Brunning R, Good RA: Congenital neutropenia: In vitro growth of colonies mimicking the disease. Proc Natl Acad Sci, USA, 70:669–672, 1973

39. Zucher-Franklin D, L'Esperance P, Good RA: Congenital neutropenia: An intrinsic cell defect demonstrated by electron microscopy of soft agar colonies. Blood 49:425–436, 1977

40. Miller ME: Pathology of chemotaxis and random mobility. Semin Hematol 12:59–82, 1975

41. Snyderman R, Pike MC: Disorders of leukocyte chemotaxis. Pediatr Clin North Am 24:377–393, 1977

42. Miller ME, Oski FA, Harris MB: Lazy leukocyte syndrome. Lancet 1:665–669, 1971

43. Boxer LA, Hedley-Whyte ET, Stossal T: Neutrophil actin dysfunction and abnormal neutrophil behavior. N Engl J Med 291:1093–1099, 1974

44. Johnston RB Jr, Newman SL: Chronic granulomatous disease. Pediatr Clin North Am 24:365–376, 1977

45. Baehner RL, Johnston RB Jr, Nathan DG: Comparative study of the metabolic and bactericidal characteristics of glucose-6-phosphate dehydrogenase-deficient polymorphonuclear leukocytes and leukocytes from children with chronic granulomatous disease. J Reticuloendothel Soc 12:150–169, 1972

46. McAllister J, Boxer LA, Baehner RL: Alteration of microtubule function in glutathione peroxidase deficient polymorphonuclear leukocytes. Clin Res, 1978, (in press)

47. Oliver JM, Berlin RD, Baehner RL, et al: Mechanisms of micro-

Index

Index

117